HIGHWAY
TO HEALTH

A NOTE FROM THE TEAM AT THE CHIROPRACTIC PHYSICIANS CENTER

"First of all, we want to thank the patients we've been privileged to serve over the years. We are blessed to see your health and lives transform in front of us. Most of our patients come to Dr. Barlow and Dr. Mackey as a "last resort." We see our clinic as the most advanced in the healthcare industry because of tools like the brain-body-gut detox program, brain-based technology, and lab tests such as Chem 77, Cyrex array #2, Cyrex array #5, and Enterolab. Identifying our patients' metabolic and autoimmune disorders validates they are not lazy, crazy, or chronic complainers. They are individuals who need help. If you are living with chronic health issues, please read this book in its entirety. If Dr. Barlow accepts you as a patient, we all look forward to seeing your life transform.

Secondly, we want to thank Dr. Barlow and Dr. Mackey. We love getting to work for you both. Our work environment doesn't feel like work, it feels like family. We don't take for granted working for a doctor who trains other doctors all over the world to do what he does here. Dr. Barlow could have kept his neurological methods to him-self, but instead he chose to train other doctors so they, too, could optimize their patients' lives. To work for doctors who truly care about their patients' health is empowering. We are blessed to be a part of your life and witness all you do for your patients and for us."

—Sandy Gann, Nikki Kennedy, Forrest Tate, and Marie Satterwhite (Dr. Barlow's Office Staff)

TESTIMONIALS OF HEALING

"Before meeting Dr. Barlow, I would have never thought my chronic pain, focus, and anxiety issues had to do with what I was eating. After reading his first book, *License to Heal: What To Do When Traditional Medicine Has Failed*, I realized there was a connection between my brain and gut. Both were influencing the way I felt. I went on Dr. Barlow's ten week detox, cut gluten out of my diet, and started doing exercises to reprogram my brain. After two weeks, I noticed a difference in how I felt. Eventually, my hip and back pain went away. Now I'm sleeping better and my focus is sharper than ever. I can't thank Dr. Barlow and his staff enough for helping me have a better quality of life. I feel amazing at the age of 52!"

—Randall Chesnutt

"Before the age of thirty I had chronic back and stomach issues, cystic acne, chronic fatigue, and many other ailments. I'd been to several doctors with little success. I saw some progress but never felt completely better. I had a couple head injuries when I was younger but had no idea they affected my gut. Dr. Barlow was the first doctor to address my brain, body, and gut simultaneously which is why I've seen such an improvement in my health. I can now eat without pain. For the first time since I was a kid, I feel like my gut is completely healed. To Dr. Barlow and your amazing staff, thank you for all of your support in improving my health."

—Toni Bubb

"When I first came into Dr. Barlow's office, I had tremendous back pain so bad that I could barely walk. I had seen his advertisement on tv and thought I would give him a try. When I got there, I was expecting to get put on a table and get my back popped and stretched like a rubber band, then to be turned loose to hope for the best. But it wasn't anything like I expected. First, he did an evaluation of what I had going on. Then did an X-ray and explained to me how he could fix the problem. I was skeptical at first, but I had already decided that I wasn't having surgery, so it was worth a try. Little did I know that after using their state-of-the-art equipment for several weeks my back would be 100 percent better. He also ran several tests and found out I had neuropathy in my feet and a leaky gut. My test results revealed that I cannot digest gluten and that had contributed to a lot of my issues. He helped me with that also. Seeing Dr. Barlow has been a blessing to me for my back and my overall health. He is straight up with you and genuinely wants to fix your problem—not just patch it up. Dr. Barlow and his friendly staff are top notch! I am a satisfied customer and would highly recommend Dr. Barlow."

—Garner Chaffin

"On October 16, 2020 I had a stroke. It affected my right leg, arm, and hand to such a degree that I could hardly walk, use my arm or hand, and experienced terrible "brain fog". On October 26, 2020, other doctors prescribed physical & occupational therapy three days a week for eight weeks. This helped to some degree, but the therapy on my right leg was so intense that my sciatic nerve began to give me lots of pain. I stopped the therapy and was in bed most of the time. Only by God's grace, I made it through to February 2021 but I knew I had to find a doctor that could help me. My husband and I had heard of Dr. Barlow and we had seen his commercials on television. I called his office for an evaluation, saw him immediately on February 8, 2021, and was on my way to relief and healing.

I didn't know anything about a stroke! My daughter went online and found out that the first thing a stroke victim needs is oxygen. I was never even given oxygen! That's the first thing Dr. Barlow started me on ... riding an exercise bike & breathing oxygen. Within three days my head felt better and the 'brain fog' was lifting. Dr. Barlow's program for the brain is amazing! My first brain map showed damage from the stroke and it wasn't good. However, after three months of therapy for my brain, my next map showed amazing results. Over the next three months there was even more good improvement. Now, I am back to teaching my Sunday School class again! Dr. Barlow thought my program would take nine to twelve months and possibly up to two years. But after only eight months, my sciatic nerve is behaving itself! If you have a stroke, see Dr. Barlow at once! Dr. Barlow is a doctor who cares, wants you to get better, and tries his best to see that you do!"

—Nina Byers

"I have nothing but praise for Dr. Barlow. In late 2020, I was unable to stand or walk for ten minutes or move or take a deep breath without pain. I went to several medical doctors and spine specialists and was told that they couldn't really help, but instead offered short-term relief with shots in the back and pain killers. I *did* take a set of shots to be able to move but knew that if I continued that route, in a short time, it would be worse and I would be mostly in a wheelchair because the shots were only covering up the root cause. Dr. Barlow was recommended, so my daughter made an appointment for me. What a difference! While other doctors would never touch me, Dr. Barlow spent more than an hour examining me and running tests. When he got through, he said that if I was willing to follow his orders, he could help me. I jumped at the chance and I'm *so* glad I did. I went through four months of intense therapy, plus I changed my diet. Now, about eight months later, I can walk two whole miles a day and do pretty much whatever I want— *plus*, fifty pounds came off! No matter what I had done before, my weight wouldn't budge. I have nothing but good things to say for Dr. Barlow's office staff also. Thank you and God bless you, Dr. Barlow; *you gave me my life back*!"

—Sheila S.

"I first came to Dr. Barlow because I was having extreme numbness and tingling in my feet. I was waking up three or more times a night to put my feet in hot water to get relief. I had gone to numerous specialists and no one could tell me what was wrong. I went through nerve conduction studies where the results showed I did *not* have neuropathy. I couldn't ride in a vehicle hardly any distance at all without major stiffness and pain. Also, I have suffered with a lot of gastric problems, and never understood why as no one could give me answers. I prayed and prayed about what to do and was led to The Chiropractic Physicians Center and Dr. Barlow. When I got there, Dr. Barlow did an extensive exam and X-rays that showed I had a leaky gut which was causing my severe abdominal pain, among other things. I started his detox program and within three days of the detox, my gastric problems completely ended. I also lost eighteen pounds during the detox. Recently, I rode from Booneville, MS to Orange Beach, AL and never had pain or even got stiff. It was a miracle! What impressed me the most with Dr. Barlow was on the first visit he told me he wasn't going to treat the problem; he was here to find and treat the *cause* of the problem. I am now sleeping soundly, not stiff, and my energy levels are unreal! I feel like a whole new person. Anytime I have had additional problems he acknowledges it immediately. I can't sing his praise enough! I highly recommend Dr. Barlow to everyone. The doctors and staff are wonderful and Dr. Barlow has completely changed my life!"

—Diane Rowland

"I started seeing Dr. Barlow for pain and stiffness in my right knee. He found the problem to be my lower back pinching a nerve. My balance was terrible, and I had almost no mobility. After three weeks of therapy, the pain went away, and I started to regain mobility. I have improved steadily over time. I also did the nutrition program and lost thirty-five pounds. I highly recommend Dr. Barlow and his staff. They are my best option."

—Ricky Moffett

"Before I started seeing Dr. Barlow, I was at a pain level of eight to nine every day and night, even with the 800 mg of Ibuprofen I was taking every day. I have been to other doctors about my knee pain with no improvement. Dr. Barlow was the first doctor to even take X-rays of my knees. I really started to see improvement by day three of my program. Now, I have been coming to Dr. Barlow's office for two months and I continue to have improvement after every therapy visit. My knees are definitely better and I am not taking any medication. The staff is the best I have ever seen. The clinic has a very comfortable and relaxing environment. I cannot say enough good things about Dr. Barlow!"

—Donald Stegall

"I started with Dr. Barlow in 2005 after suffering whiplash in a car accident. While I had gone to other chiropractors over the years for lower back pain, I immediately noticed that Dr. Barlow's clinic and staff were doing things a bit differently than any doctors I had encountered before. I soon found that Dr. Barlow was on the cutting edge of providing the best in chiropractic health care. Over the years, I've seen Dr. Barlow, his associate chiropractors, and staff continue to learn and introduce the kinds of innovations that really impact the health of their patients. I have nothing but gratitude for all the ways Dr. Barlow's clinic has kept me on my feet and made my life almost completely pain-free. There is so much more I could say but I will leave it at this. Thank you, Dr. Barlow, Dr. Mackey, and all of your staff—past and present."

—Robert Kilpatrick

Dr. Andy Barlow, DC, DACNB, FACFN

HIGHWAY TO HEALTH

THE ROAD TO OVERCOMING DEPRESSION, ANXIETY, INSOMNIA, AND CHRONIC PAIN THROUGH THE GUT-BRAIN CONNECTION

BARLOW
BRAIN
& BODY
INSTITUTE
PUBLISHING

POWERED BY THRONE PUBLISHING

ISBN Softcover: 978-1-949550-67-2
Ebook ISBN: 978-1-949550-68-9

Printed in the United States of America.

Lead Writer: Kelli Kissack
Publishing Manager: Alle Byeseda

Although the author and publisher have made every effort to ensure that the information and advice in this book were correct and accurate at press time, the author and publisher do not assume and hereby disclaim any liability to any party for any loss, damage, or disruption caused from acting upon the information in this book or by errors or omissions, whether such errors or omissions result from negligence, accident, or any other cause.

Barlow Brain & Body Institute
266 County Road 506
Shannon, MS 38868
www.barlowbrainandbody.com

TABLE OF CONTENTS

PART TWO
PAIN, GUT, AND THE BRAIN

PART THREE
MOVING FORWARD TODAY

DEDICATION

First, I want to dedicate this book to my wife, Faye. You have changed my life in every way one human being can change another human being's life. I want to thank you for thirty-plus years of unwavering love, patience, support, and sacrifice, along with six years of weeknight and weekend studying for my diploma and fellowship in Functional Neurology.

You not only tolerate, but champion my weeknight and weekend studying of the latest medical journals. You encourage me as I travel and teach other doctors through the Barlow Brain & Body Institute. Faye, I am genuinely in awe of you, and you are my everything.

Secondly, I would like to dedicate this book to my mom, Peggy White, my business partner and son, Dr. Matt Mackey, and his wife, Tammy. My daughters, Jennifer Mackey and Karla Swanigan. My grandchildren, Zachary Roberts, Evan Swanigan, Caleb Mackey, Charlotte Mackey, and Colbie Mackey. A massive shout out to my brother, Randy Barlow, and his wife, Angel, and my brother, TJ White, and his wife, Jill. Last but certainly not least, my two fabulous nieces, Lela and Delilah White.

Thirdly, I want to dedicate this book to all the people who are currently suffering due to our broken health care system. If the "system" has failed, ignored, or overlooked you, I understand your frustration, and I want you to see this book as the turning point in your life.

Fourthly, I dedicate *Highway To Health* to every health-care professional who is a continual learner, attending advanced seminars, and striving to improve the quality of your patients' lives. Never stop learning. The world needs you.

FOREWORD

The first time we arrived at Dr. Barlow's office in Tupelo, Mississippi, from Raleigh, North Carolina, we were amazed not only at the packed parking lot at his office but also at the variety of states on the license plates on the cars. As we walked through the front doors, we saw happy patients receiving treatments and conversing with each other. We spent some time talking with them, and one after another told us about the monumental improvements they were experiencing in their lives. Each wanted to tell their particular story about how they had seen so many other doctors but did not receive significant results until they had started treatment with Dr. Andy Barlow, DC, DACNB, FACFN.

Nearly ten years and dozens of trips and class modules later, we continue to learn the latest in cutting-edge treatment protocols from Dr. Barlow to optimize the health of the patients in our own practice. With his unquenchable thirst for knowledge and daily studies, he brings unique insight and solutions for complex chronic, neurological, and metabolic problems of patients, presenting them in an easy-to-understand way.

It is rare that you come across a brilliant mind like Dr. Barlow's. It is even rarer for that awesome mentor and sage to become a treasured friend as he has become for us. We have enjoyed meeting doctors not just from all over the United States but from around the world while training with Dr. Barlow at the Barlow Brain & Body Institute.

How gratifying it is for us to confidently and clearly explain the root cause of our patients' frustrating, nagging, and debilitating health challenges and then to map out the course of their care to optimize their health so they can enjoy their life again.

We know that our patients are back to their favorite activities whether sports, shopping, traveling, or playing with their grandkids, all thanks to our coaching and studies with Dr. Barlow. What are you missing out on? The clarity of direction provided by Dr. Barlow's knowledge and experience can give you the life you always thought you should be living. We have been practicing for more than three decades and studied with incredible minds in the United States and abroad, but none has created the certainty and transformation in our practice and our own lives as Dr. Barlow has done for us and the patients we treat.

We always learn from Dr. Barlow's insights, and we are sure you will too.

Dr. Shelly Dranko, DC, DOM
& Dr. Jack Gorlesky, DC, L.Ac

INTRODUCTION

Patients often ask me, "Where are you from?" When I say, "Pontotoc, Mississippi," they are usually surprised that a doctor from a small, southern town coaches other doctors all over the United States. *Highway to Health* is my response to this reaction. This book shows my readers how a "small-town chiropractor" helps patients overcome depression, anxiety, insomnia, and chronic pain through the gut-brain connection.

Highway to Health also offers hope and education. Being a board-certified Chiropractic Neurologist and a Fellow of the American College of Functional Neurology equips me to go deeper than other medical or chiropractic doctors. There may be a solution to your problem that traditional medical doctors haven't presented to you.

Highway to Health teaches my readers what they can do in the space between the initial and final stages of chronic medical issues. Many of my patients have gone from doctor to doctor trying to solve their problems. Sadly, by the time their condition reaches a stage advanced enough for a clinical diagnosis, they are often already in a disease state for issues like Rheumatoid Arthritis, Multiple Sclerosis (MS), or Amyotrophic Lateral Sclerosis (ALS). If you are in danger of going down this road of destruction, *Highway to Health* exists to educate you about specific tests that can help determine if you are in a disease state and what we can do to slow it down (or even stop it).

I have made it my life's mission to provide effective, in-office solutions for my patients near and far, and I firmly believe educated patients make better decisions about their health. I have seen people change their lives by simply taking ownership of their health journey, and I know you can make this change too.

> *"Let the rest do whatever, while you do whatever it takes."*

—GRANT CARDONE

PART ONE

STARTING AGAIN

CHAPTER ONE

WHEN I STARTED AGAIN

*"The further a society drifts from the truth,
the more they will hate those that speak it."*

—Selwyn Duke

AN IMPROVED PARADIGM

Imagine spending four years attending chiropractic college, practicing as a chiropractor for five years, and then dedicating six years to studying for a diploma and fellowship in functional neurology, only to discover I still didn't have the answers I needed to heal the person I love most, my wife, Faye. That was an eye-opening realization for a doctor who prided himself on being current with the latest medical research. It was also very motivating. For several years, Faye had struggled with her thyroid. She also had the autoimmune-based skin problem of vitiligo. While these issues didn't prevent her from doing the things she wanted to do, I knew there had to be underlying causes that weren't being addressed.

Yet I didn't just lack answers for Faye's condition. There were patients coming into my clinic for neurological treatment that clearly had autoimmune struggles too. I was helping them improve their neurological issues, but I knew to achieve true health and vitality and optimize their recovery, they must be set free from the autoimmune dysfunction that held them back. I had a choice to make: either ignore it and continue treating everything like a neurological problem, turning a blind eye to the metabolic aspect of health care or face the reality that I needed to ask different questions to solve these health problems. Ultimately, my desire to help Faye and my patients sent me back to a place with which I was familiar, school. I chose to return to the Kharrazian Institute, this time to study functional medicine. I knew someone out there had the answers I sought, and I was determined to find them.

My functional medicine studies led me to ask new questions, discover new philosophies, and finally uncover the key I'd been seeking. I'd studied the brain extensively while completing my fellowship in functional neurology through the Carrick Institute, but my true "eureka" moment came when I learned of the existence of the brain-gut connection. Talk about a light bulb moment! The brain and the gut (essentially, the digestive system) are connected by the vagus nerve (known as "the wanderer"). It's the longest and most complex of the twelve pairs of cranial nerves. It acts as a superhighway of connectivity between the brain and the gut, and vice versa.

I learned that most chronic neurological disorders actually originate in the gut first then manifest in the brain. Here exists a superhighway of communication, connectedness, and a relationship between the gut and the brain that I'd known about before but never really understood. Here was the answer. My desire to help Faye with her autoimmune condition turned into an epic journey of learning and re-arranging all the health paradigms I'd previously known, and this gut-brain connection was the key I needed to help my patients unlock their full potential for health, healing, and vitality.

Through my studies of functional medicine and the gut-brain connection, I began to learn about leaky gut, a digestive condition that allows undigested proteins, bacteria, toxins, and gluten to leak through the intestinal wall into the sterile bloodstream. I discovered that this seemingly simple condition can lead to an inflammatory cascade and trigger an autoimmune reaction in the brain, gut, and body. My paradigm continued to expand and shift as I realized that Faye's autoimmune conditions were likely being triggered by our diet and environment. I also learned that gluten, a protein found in wheat, barley, and rye, was one of the most vicious culprits in causing leaky-gut inflammation as well as autoimmunity because most people genetically cannot digest the modern forms of gluten so common in our food.

During my studies, I was introduced to Enterolab, a lab that tests for the gluten gene as well as the celiac gene and malabsorption issues. Tests results show a) if you carry the gene(s) for gluten intolerance and b) whether the gluten gene(s) were turned on and currently active, potentially damaging your tissues and organs. I encouraged Faye to take this test, and I decided to take it as well to be a supportive husband, of course. When the results came back, I was shocked. Not only did Faye have the turned-on gene for gluten intolerance, but so did I, only my symptoms hadn't manifested yet. Talk about a surprise! I thought I was being a hero by supporting my wife, and it turned out I too had a gluten sensitivity disorder.

This was another turning point in my journey both as a doctor and as a person seeking vibrant, long-lasting health. I had a choice to make. Would I ignore the science and the lab results and continue living my life the way I always had? Or would I get ahead of this inflammatory process before it turned into a potential autoimmune condition and address it by radically changing my diet and lifestyle? Faye and I had to ask ourselves the same question I now ask all of my patients, "How far are we willing to go? What are we willing to do to fix this problem for good, optimize our health, and live life to its fullest?"

We wanted to be well and decided we were willing to do what it took to ensure that would happen. Once I understood the powerful connection between the brain and the gut via the vagus nerve, major changes began to happen. We needed to optimize our brain function and heal our guts. This meant making some major lifestyle changes.

For starters, we completely eliminated gluten from our diet. We also embarked on a ten-week program commonly called the brain and body detox. These two changes kick-started the healing of our leaky guts and helped decrease the inflammation in our bodies. Faye is a wonderful cook, and she immediately got to work learning how to make all of our family's favorite foods using gluten-free flour. Like everyone who undertakes a major lifestyle change, we went through our share of learning experiences as we adjusted to our new normal.

One of my favorite stories from this season involves Faye's first experiments making homemade, gluten-free biscuits. She and I were both surprised when they came out looking (and tasting) like hockey pucks rather than fluffy, flaky Southern-style biscuits. Now, we can laugh about the hockey puck biscuits, but like anyone learning something new, we made lots of mistakes. The difference is that we didn't let it discourage us. We learned from those mistakes, fixed them, and kept moving forward, and so can you.

By reading Faye and my story, I hope you see that I'm not sharing anything in this book that my family and I aren't also willing to do. Today, both of Faye's autoimmune conditions are in complete remission. My gluten intolerance disorder never manifested symptoms, and today I live a vibrant, healthy life. I play racquetball several days per week, see hundreds of patients each year at my clinic in Tupelo, Mississippi, and coach doctors nationally and internationally through my Barlow Brain & Body Institute. I am passionate about the health of the gut and the brain because my family and I have personally experienced the life-changing benefits of this program.

Speaking of my clinic, once Faye and I experienced such amazing results, I began to implement these new strategies with my patients. Instead of only treating neurological issues, I began to treat the gut and the brain simultaneously. In addition to the in-depth neurological exams I'd always done, I began implementing new tools like the Enterolab tests and in-depth blood work with such organizations as Cyrex and LabCorp to uncover the metabolic root causes of my patients' problems. I knew we were on the right track when we began seeing chronic pain patients go from a pain level of seven or eight down to a one or two. I also began seeing a dramatic improvement in people suffering from anxiety, depression, and insomnia.

We'll talk more about why this happened later in the book. For now, consider a car. A car can appear in perfect condition on the outside, but it won't start or run if the gas tank is empty, the spark plugs are missing, or the battery is dead. That's how the body works too. The inside runs the outside, and for the inside to be truly healthy, the gut-brain connection must be addressed.

The bottom line is that brain-based disorders and leaky gut syndrome are not going away. If you or someone you love is struggling with chronic pain or an autoimmune condition, the purpose of this book is to let you know there may be help, hope, and a future for you. However, if you want vibrant health and a hopeful future, you must take responsibility for your life. Each year, I see hundreds of people suffering from what they believe are permanent conditions. They've been told by traditional doctors that nothing can be done and they simply must "learn to live with it."

I'm here to say, "No, that's not necessarily true!" This is your wake-up call. If a doctor treats the brain or gut, they usually treat them separately. I've learned if they are simultaneously treated together, you can achieve stratospheric results.

Your health, and therefore your life, can change for the better, and the first step toward healing is understanding that your future is in your hands. These things can be changed if you decide to make the change. Your life, your purpose, and the things you have to offer the world are too important to be held back by chronic pain and autoimmune dysfunction. If you've been told by a mainstream medical doctor that there's no hope for you, remember something is only impossible until it's done for the first time. The only thing stopping you from going from where you are to where you want to be is what you're not willing to do. That's the limiting factor.

CHAPTER TWO

THE STANDARD AMERICAN DIET

"You'll never change your life until you change something you do daily. The secret to success is found in your daily routine."

—John Maxwell

WINNING THE WRONG GAME

Have you ever heard of the standard American diet (SAD)? It's fitting this phrase carries the acronym SAD because that's literally how it makes millions of Americans feel. To truly understand the genesis of the SAD, let's think back a few generations and consider the food our ancestors ate. Most of our grandparents consumed things that grew in the ground, on a tree, or that they killed. They ate real, unprocessed foods, fruits and vegetables, meat that they raised or hunted, eggs from chickens in their backyard, and healthy fats like butter and lard. If they ate bread, it was made at home from flour that was not milled from hybridized, pesticide-laced wheat. In short, they ate real, unmodified, unprocessed food. Now let's compare the diet of our ancestors with the diet of most twenty-first-century Americans.

Today, convenience is king. Fast food rules. Most food comes packaged in a bag, box, or plastic wrapper. Very few people grow their own vegetables and fruit and even fewer raise their own meat. It's easier than ever to buy Wonder Bread, Pop Tarts, or potato chips at the supermarket. The majority of meat animals are raised on commercial farms and fed a diet of GMO corn, soy, and wheat. Eggs are produced in huge factory farms where the hens are fed—you guessed it—GMO corn, soy, and hybridized wheat.

Let's take a look at what a regular, American child eats on the SAD:

> SAD breakfast: low nutritional value pastries, sugary cereal, and milk or orange juice.
>
> SAD lunch: low nutritional value processed food because it's cheap at school.
>
> SAD dinner: low nutritional value sandwich, potato chips, and soda.

The average adult's diet is no different, consisting of fast food, processed food (comes in a bag or box), and soda or, even worse, diet soda. The scarier news is gluten is laced into nearly all of this processed food. Today's food lacks the vitamins, minerals, and nutritional value of the food of our ancestors' era. It's higher in calories, lower in nutrition, and full of more inflammatory factors than ever before. If you don't believe me, look at pictures of the average American family from the 1970s and 1980s. Maybe one person was overweight. Today, one person is likely trim and fit, and everyone else in the picture is fat, overweight, or morbidly obese. We've traded nutrition for convenience, real food for genetically modified and/or hybridized replacements, and quality for quantity. The worst part is people don't understand what they're doing wrong because they've done it wrong for so long that wrong has become "normal." So what's the result of this diabolical diet change in America?

There are three major issues stemming from the low-quality, high caloric nature of SAD. We'll look at each of them briefly in this chapter and then explore in-depth solutions to these problems in subsequent chapters.

PROBLEM #1: GLUTEN SENSITIVITY

Gluten, a protein composite found in wheat, exists in nearly every kind of processed food available at fast food restaurants and on grocery shelves today. The reason modern-day gluten is a problem for our guts (digestive systems) is that modern wheat has been hybridized (Different varieties of wheat have been cross-bred to produce new, modern varieties.) to increase harvest yields and maximize resistance to pests and disease. Unfortunately, our bodies don't have the right enzymes to digest these new varieties. When we eat gluten, undigested protein leaks into the bloodstream where our bodies recognize it as a foreign invader, cueing up our immune system to attack and kill it. This process is like sandpaper rubbing on the gut barrier, similar to a leak in your roof. It starts small but has huge long-term effects. This inflammatory reaction happens every time an "invasion" happens, which for Americans eating the SAD is at least three times per day. Imagine if a robber broke into your home three times per day. You would eventually get tired of fighting off the invader, right? That's what happens to our immune system too. Our body gets tired of fighting and gives up, resulting in autoimmune conditions, fatigue, brain fog, insomnia, depression, anxiety, chronic pain, and so on.

Gluten sensitivity is an exaggerated immune response to gluten that leads to an inflammatory reaction throughout the brain, gut, and body and can lead to an autoimmune response, thereby, causing the immune system to attack, break down, and eventually destroy the brain, gut, and body tissue. The literature recognizes it as a trigger in cognitive impairment, dementia, psychiatric disorders (e.g., anxiety, depression, bipolar disorders, obsessive-compulsive disorders, autism), movement disorders, general neurological impairment, ataxia (lack of muscle control and coordination), restless leg syndrome, neuropathy (numbness, tingling, pins and needles in hands and/or feet), myoclonus (sudden, brief involuntary twitching or jerking of a muscle or group of muscles), myopathy (muscle weakness), multiple sclerosis, cerebellum disease (responsible for controlling gait and muscle coordination), neuromuscular disease (the most common sign of these diseases is muscle weakness), and migraine headaches. As you can see, gluten sensitivity can negatively impact almost everything regarding the nervous system as well as your thyroid gland, joints, and skin.

PROBLEM #2: INFLAMMATORY PROCESSES

Think of inflammation as a fire in your body. If you had a fire in your house, you would put that fire out completely before repairing the damage. This is similar to how inflammation affects the body. It's important to note that not all inflammation is bad. In fact, it serves a great purpose for acute injuries like a sprained ankle. If you twist your ankle playing basketball, inflammation draws the healing processes to the area and starts repairing the damage. However, chronic inflammation is not good. Chronic inflammation, which can be triggered by a variety of dietary or environmental factors (especially the SAD), acts as a river of hot, molten lava going through your body. It's destructive, creates all sorts of secondary problems, and must be eliminated before the body can begin to heal itself.

If you're curious about your body's level of chronic inflammation, here are three of the best indicators. These markers can easily be identified through blood work; however, they will likely not be on the blood panels ordered by your general practitioner. You will need to specifically ask for these markers to be tested.

1) A1C: This should be below 5.6. Levels above 5.6 indicate pre-diabetes and major inflammation.
2) C-Reactive Protein (CRP): This should be below 3 mg/L.
3) Homocysteine: This should be between 5–7 mmol/L.

Let's look at how chronic inflammation manifests in different areas of the body.

1. Body: This causes the tissue destruction of muscles, joints, and ligaments, which leads to chronic pain.
2. Brain: This triggers anxiety, depression, insomnia, and lack of focus and attention.
3. Gut: This manifests as gastroesophageal reflux disease (GERD), irritable bowel syndrome (IBS), bloating, distention, malabsorption disorder, leaky gut, and more.

There's not an exact way of predicting how inflammation will affect each person, but we know it attacks the weakest area of the body first. An invading army doesn't start at the thickest part of the city wall. No, they aim for the wooden gate because it's the weakest spot. The same is true of inflammation. It finds the weakest area of your body and settles there first.

PROBLEM #3: BLOOD SUGAR DYSREGULATION

The SAD is high in sugar and carbohydrates, and consumption of these sugary, highly processed foods drives up blood sugar levels. This poor diet carries a one-two punch: a) inflammation and b) diabetes. Blood sugar or glucose comes from the food you eat and is your body's main source of energy. Your blood carries glucose to all of your body's cells to be converted to energy, but too much sugar in the blood can have disastrous effects. A range of 85–99 mg/dL is considered optimal. Blood glucose from 100–125 mg/dL is considered insulin resistant (the precursor to diabetes), and anything over 126 mg/dL is officially Type 2 diabetes. The higher your blood sugar levels are, the higher your inflammation levels. These two markers go hand-in-hand. Processed food containing gluten combined with a high-carb diet creates an inflammatory cascade that drives up blood sugar and triggers inflammatory processes in the body. This ultimately causes long-term damage to the brain, body, and gut.

As you can see, diet is incredibly important to one's overall health. One of my favorite sayings is, "Man's food kills, and God's food heals." The sad part is that most people have no idea how crucial their diet is to achieving vibrant health and long-term wellness. Why? If a lie is told long enough, people start to believe it. Many of us were never taught that gluten-containing, carb-laden processed foods are bad for us. It's normal, it's the way we were raised, and most everyone is doing it. Yet the research is devastatingly clear: the SAD is destroying our bodies and our health. We can't fulfill our

God-given potential if we're slowly killing ourselves with these foods. If you're having chronic health problems but not addressing your diet, it's like having a giant hole in the roof and only worrying about emptying the buckets of water on the floor. To make things better, you first have to stop making them worse.

TWO SCHOOLS OF THOUGHT

When it comes to treating chronic health problems, two schools of thought rule the day.

1. The gut and brain are completely separate from each other and the rest of the body, therefore, treat them separately. The gut and brain are interconnected through the vagus nerve, therefore acknowledge the latest scientific research confirming this and treat them together.
2. Also, treat the whole body as an inclusive system that's supposed to work together and exist harmoniously.

Before I knew better, I belonged to the first camp. Now that both I've learned the truth and the scientific research is clear, I've strongly staked my flag in the second one. The brain, body, and gut make up a whole, complete system that works together. If we want to improve chronic health issues like pain or autoimmune conditions, we must treat these parts of the whole simultaneously.

Through working with patients at my clinic, spending hundreds of hours reading the latest medical journals, and walking my personal journey of healing, I've realized three fundamental truths that explain why diet is so critical to health:

1. Gluten is the most toxic food product you can put in your body.
2. Today's processed food lacks the total essential vitamins and minerals that our bodies need to function optimally. The SAD has minimal, if any, nutritional value, and consequently, the majority of Americans are walking around with serious vitamin and mineral deficiencies.
3. What you put in your mouth is either going to heal you or kill you.

I state these truths so confidently because I've tested hundreds of patients at my clinic and reviewed the test results myself. There are three main metabolic tests I use to understand where the cascade of inflammation is originating. These tests reveal three crucial things:

1. Whether the patient carries the gene(s) for gluten sensitivity or celiac, known as the HLA-DQB1 gene;
2. Whether they have a leaky gut; and
3. Whether they have any underlying autoimmune conditions lurking beneath the surface, and if so, which area of the body has been negatively affected.

When it comes to gluten sensitivity genes, you can carry zero, one, or two of them. If you have none of the genes, it's unlikely for gluten sensitivity to affect you. If you carry one gene, you are less predisposed to having gluten sensitivity than if you carry two genes. Having two gluten genes is the most serious scenario. Out of the hundreds of patients I've tested in my clinic, only two patients have had no genes for gluten sensitivity, and the majority of people carry two. These genes behave like light switches. They can be activated by environmental factors, and, once active, they are very difficult to turn off. It's not surprising that consuming gluten has a high probability of turning them on.

The other problem with gluten is that it's addictive. Why? When it crosses the blood-brain barrier into the brain, it transforms into a gluteomorphin (a morphine like morphine) and docks on your brain's opioid receptor site, known as the nucleus accumbens. You read it right; once gluten enters your brain, your brain receives it as an addictive substance and produces essentially the same response as if you ingested heroin or morphine.

SETTING YOURSELF FREE

By this point in the book, you may be thinking, "Dr. Barlow, how can this all be true? How are my morning toast and cereal the root cause of my acid reflux and chronic pain?" Do you remember what I said earlier in the chapter? Just because we've been told a lie for a long time doesn't make it true. Whole-wheat cereal is not good for you. Sugary cakes and pastries are not harmless treats. Fast food isn't a more convenient way to eat dinner. Just because everyone else is doing it doesn't make it any less harmful to us. Look at your coworkers, church members, and family. Are they healthy or overweight? Full of energy or constantly fatigued? Do they suffer from anxiety, depression, headaches, or insomnia? Just because these problems are common doesn't make them normal. There's a better way to live.

As a friend and doctor, I ask that you please commit to reading the rest of this book. Answers and hope are ahead. We all have an expiration date, so isn't it time to get our acts together? If you're on the fence, think about it this way: you've done it your way up until now, and it's not working. Now, consider an approach that's scientifically proven to work. Start a new chapter in your life today. Your legacy is too valuable to be diminished by chronic health problems. Be responsible to your family; they want to see you vivacious, full of energy, and cognitively healthy too. We can't expect the government, Big Pharma or our insurance companies to fix our issues for us. It's time to commit to your health and vitality.

I ask all my patients, "How far do you want to go?" Now, I'm asking you the same question. How far are you willing to go to reclaim your health?

CHAPTER THREE

THE BRAIN-GUT CONNECTION

"I am not a product of my circumstances.
I am a product of my decisions."

—Steven Covey

YOUR BREAKTHROUGH UNDERSTANDING

The first step to reclaiming your health is understanding the amazing machine that is your body and how it works. It's not a bunch of individual organs operating independently of each other. Instead, it's an interconnected system working together holistically through constant communication from the brain to the body, the body to the brain, the brain to the gut, and the gut to the brain.

Many of us instinctively understand that our brains and bodies communicate back and forth. For example, you can see a glass of water sitting on the counter and pick it up. Your brain (frontal lobe) sends a signal to your hand, and you pick up the glass. In return, your hand sends a signal back to your brain (parietal lobe) noting the weight, shape, and condensation on the glass. This action is possible because of the brain-body feedback loop. The brain sends a neurological signal to your hand, and in return your hand sends a neurological signal back to your brain. This is the part of the nervous system responsible for executing voluntary actions like picking up a glass or throwing a ball across the yard.

However, there's a whole other part of the system that's easy to forget, the autonomic nervous system. Though we don't often think about it, we're in big trouble if it stops functioning. This ultra-important system controls all of the involuntary actions necessary for living such as our heart beating, lungs breathing, and the subject of this chapter, digestion.

To understand our digestion, we look to one of the main divisions of our autonomic nervous system known as the enteric nervous system, a mesh-like system of neurons that governs the duties of the gastrointestinal tract. We can easily forget about this incredible system because we don't make it function by thinking about it. Instead, the brain and gut talk back and forth on their own about the complex process of digestion.

Many people don't realize that the outside world is what's inside our guts. We ingest food that travels to our stomach, and the stomach sends a signal to the brain saying the food has arrived and it's time to release hydrochloric acid, the substance that breaks down food in the stomach. Next, the broken-down food reaches the small intestine where it encounters epithelial cells. These epithelial cells form a single-layer barrier between what's inside your gut and what gets through that protective lining, which eventually ends up in your bloodstream. Along the way, your brain communicates with your gallbladder, signaling it to contract and release bile. It also talks with the liver and pancreas, perfectly timing the release of critical digestive enzymes that break fats, proteins, and carbohydrates into smaller components your body can easily digest. The small intestine is where your food is broken down, assimilated into your bloodstream, and absorbed, whereas the large intestine's main function is taking water out of your feces before it's eliminated from the body. The large intestine is also home to our microbiome, which we will talk about in a later chapter. As this is all happening, your brain is controlling the speed at which your food moves through your gut, which is known as "gut motility." When the system is healthy, this is all done automatically without our thinking about it.

The main superhighway of communication between the brain and the gut is the vagus nerve, one of the biggest, fattest nerves in the body. The technical term for a nerve like this is "highly myelinated," which simply means it's heavily coated with a thick layer of myelin, basically an insulating layer that forms around nerves. It's made of protein and fatty substances and acts as a conductor for signals sent throughout the nervous system. The more myelinated a nerve, the faster it can send signals to and from the brain.

You may be thinking, "Dr. Barlow, this information is all well and good, but why does it matter to me that my brain, body, and gut communicate with one another?" To illustrate just how vitally important this topic is to your health, think about your heart. Why is it important that your brain and heart have a healthy, open highway of communication? Because if they don't, your heart stops beating, and you die. Now think about your lungs. Why is it important that your lungs and brain talk back and forth effectively? Same reason, if they don't, you lose oxygen supply and expire within minutes. In fact, a person needs to breathe twenty to sixteen times per minute for optimal function because oxygen is necessary for life. Thanks to the vagus nerve, if you're not breathing as you should, a signal is sent to your brain saying, "Breathe deeply or more often so there's more oxygen supply."

Just as your heart and lung functions are necessary for staying alive, so is your digestion. Your gut health is just as important as your brain health, and the two working in sync are the key to living a healthy, vibrant life. The brain communicates with the gut for the main function of assimilating and breaking down nutrients, and we each need these vital nutrients for our brain to function and our body to heal itself. Like a conductor coordinating the intricate movements of an orchestra, our brain is the grand conductor signaling back and forth with the gut to time these important movements such as secreting hydrochloric acid and enzymatically breaking down fat, protein, and carbohydrates. The way our gut breaks down food, extracts vital nutrients, and gets those nutrients into the bloodstream is what feeds our body and brain, and all of these processes are intricately timed. If even one action happens too soon or too late, the whole process is compromised.

The brain controls and coordinates gut motility and timing mechanisms as each digestive organ signals back to the brain exactly what's happening, ensuring every movement happens on time. The gut and brain constantly communicate back and forth ensuring smooth transitions in motility to successfully break down food for absorption. If this communication fails, malabsorption issues result. Symptoms may include gastric reflux, heartburn, bloating, belching, constipation, and diarrhea. Some of my patients even tell me it feels like a brick is in their stomach.

The brain says what to do and when to do it, and the gut calls back saying, "OK, that's done, and now this is done."

The brain controls the motility (movement of food through the gut), and the gut fires back to the brain saying,

"OK, we're at this point of the process. Now we need to get ready for the next step."

Your enteric nervous system (gut) is constantly communicating with your brain saying, "Here's where the food products are, and here's the next step."

Your brain then signals which enzymes are released and how quickly it all must move through the system with the ultimate goal of successful absorption so the body gets the vital nutrients it needs to heal.

We've looked at communication between the brain and the gut; now, let's dig into the ways chronic pain, the brain, and the gut are connected. As mentioned earlier, our frontal lobe controls our movements, like picking up a glass of water. Our parietal lobe receives the sensory input from our hand to feel the weight, shape and condensation on the glass. However, that's only a fraction of the overall function of both the frontal and parietal lobes. The frontal lobe moves the body and controls focus, attention, concentration, goal setting, planning, happiness, overall emotional well-being, social interactions, impulse control, learning, and memory. Our parietal lobe both receives input from the body and helps maintain our balance and awareness of where we are in space. When our frontal lobe is malfunctioning due to chronic inflammation, blood sugar dysregulation, gluten, leaky gut, gut malabsorption issues, and/or autoimmunity, we may start to notice things such as loss of focus, attention, concentration, mental and physical fatigue, anxiety, depression, insomnia, loss of emotional control, lack of social skills, obsessive compulsive disorders, loss of the ability to learn new things, and memory loss. When our parietal lobe malfunctions, we may notice loss of sensation in our feet and hands, loss of balance, cold feet and hands, numbness and tingling in our extremities, and chronic pain syndromes like fibromyalgia. All of these issues are linked to chronic inflammation, blood sugar dysregulation, gluten, leaky gut, gut malabsorption issues, and/or autoimmunity.

The other common source of chronic pain as it relates to the gut starts with the vagus nerve. As I mentioned earlier, this nerve is a superhighway of communication, and when our brain fires a signal down to the enteric nervous system (responsible for communication in the gut), it does so via the vagus nerve. Chronic inflammation, blood sugar dysregulation, gluten, leaky gut, malabsorption issues and/or autoimmune disorders can all slow down or damage the transmission of signals between our brain and gut or body, leading to a multitude of chronic health problems like anxiety, depression, insomnia, chronic pain syndromes, memory issues, balance disorders, gastric reflux, heartburn, bloating, or constipation. But, no worries, your doctor has a prescription for every symptom above (sarcasm intended).

This reminds me of a fifty-six-year-old female who came to my office suffering from mental fatigue, anxiety, insomnia, and chronic pain all over her body. She had almost given up any hope of recovery. During our conversation, I asked about her gut function and past trauma (e.g., car accidents, sports-related injuries). She gave the usual response to gut issues: gastric reflux, constipation, bloating. Her first car accident was at age seventeen, rear impact, and the second at age thirty-five, driver's side impact. (We'll talk more about trauma and its impact on brain-gut health in the next chapter). Her neurological exam revealed cold hands and feet and sensory issues in her feet. All motor reflexes were slow, and her balance was terrible. When she put both feet together, she fell to the right in two seconds. (You should be able to hold that position for fifteen seconds.) These are just a few of the tests I performed to evaluate her frontal and parietal lobe function.

We also completed the metabolic blood work program. She had chronic inflammation, her glucose was high, her liver was not functioning properly, and she had both gluten genes and malabsorption issues. She also had two positive tissues from her Cyrex Array 5 autoimmune test as well as a leaky gut from the Cyrex Array 2. Working to rehabilitate her brain and gut function simultaneously, we began seeing improvements within four weeks. She went from a bummed-out fifty-six-year-old in constant pain to a happy, friendly person full of energy. I share her story to show that by working with your gut and brain, your body can heal and accomplish things you never dreamed it could. Now, let's go deeper into the source of chronic pain and how we treat it.

PART TWO

PAIN, GUT, AND THE BRAIN

CHAPTER FOUR

THE UNEXPECTED SOURCE OF CHRONIC PAIN

"When you stop chasing the wrong things, you give the right things a chance to catch up."

—Lolly Daskal

THE SECRET SOURCE OF PAIN

Would you be surprised if I told you the most common source of chronic pain is past trauma? Most people only think of trauma as physical, yet the truth is the brain can't distinguish between physical and psychological trauma. I almost exclusively see patients with a wide array of chronic health problems, and every single one of them has some kind of past trauma from ten to fifteen years prior, and some patients as far back as thirty or forty years. To better understand this concept, let's look at the way physical trauma affects the brain in the long-term.

Car accidents, concussions from sports-related injuries, and traumas from extreme emotional events (known as post-traumatic stress disorder or PTSD) affect the brain in similar ways. The brain is home to a type of cell known as microglial cells. They are found in the central nervous system, and their job is removing damaged neurons, infections, and other debris from the brain and spinal cord. When the brain is damaged by concussion or severe emotional trauma, these cells are turned on. Once they're on, they're very hard to turn off. When they remain chronically on, they begin damaging and destroying healthy brain cells. Studies have shown that chronic blood sugar dysregulation, chronic inflammation, and gluten can also trigger the effect.

When this happens, the frontal cortex is usually affected first. The symptoms manifest as smaller things like focus and attention disorders. If those early symptoms aren't addressed, it progresses into the next stage of anxiety, depression, insomnia, and memory disorders. If those symptoms aren't addressed, the trouble moves to the parietal lobe and manifests as chronic pain disorders.

Psychological trauma works similarly to physical trauma, which is received by the brain as emotional stress, yet the brain doesn't distinguish between physical and psychological stress. Say a woman receives a letter from the IRS: stress. Then she loses her job: stress. A loved one passes: stress. Covid hits home: stress. Stress, stress, and more stress. This psychological trauma will actually affect her physically by changing her brain function and sending stress responses down to the gut, creating problems there as well. Chronic stress is devastating to the brain, particularly the frontal lobe, because it cues the release of excess cortisol, which in turn damages the hippocampus (a complex brain structure embedded deep in the temporal lobe that plays a major role in learning and memory) and leads to memory disorders like Alzheimer's disease.

But wait, how does all of this relate to the root cause of chronic pain? When any aspect of your neurology slows down, the brain tissues get close to threshold, which simply means they fire easily, like having a hair trigger on a gun. Nerves get too close to threshold and require very little stimulation to make them fire, which leads to overactive nerve responses and manifests as chronic pain syndromes like hyperalgesia and allodynia. For someone with either of these conditions, things that shouldn't normally be painful like swiping a cotton ball over the skin or being lightly poked with a toothpick register as intense pain because their nerves fire too easily.

Chronic stress also has a drastic effect on the brain-gut connection. Think about the way people experienced stress ten thousand years ago; they had periods of intense stress, like outrunning a saber tooth tiger, and then the stressor disappeared. When a person is in a stressful, life-threatening situation, their body doesn't care about digesting food. It cares about survival. The same principle is true today. Gut motility slows down in times of stress, even chronic stress. Instead of passing through in twenty-four to forty-eight hours, food stays in the body and rots.

Yuck.

Slow digestion creates a cascade of negativity like bacterial and yeast overgrowth, gastric reflux, bloating, constipation, and so on: an entire cascade of dysfunction all because chronic stress slowed the brain down.

In summary, the brain slows down from these five things:

1) Chronic Stress
2) Past Physical or Psychological Trauma
3) Gluten Sensitivity
4) Blood Sugar Dysregulation (via the SAD)
5) Chronic Inflammation

Gluten sensitivity, blood sugar dysregulation, and trauma: what do all of these conditions have in common?

They cause chronic inflammation, and chronic inflammation affects the brain, body, and gut. Inflammation of the brain turns on the aforementioned microglial cells, which eventually slows down the brain's function. When brain function slows down, the vagus nerve doesn't fire as well, which leads to gut dysfunction.

I describe patients as a "web of dysfunction" because one, two, or all of these factors could be contributing to their chronic health problems, and very few doctors piece all of these triggers together. This is also why lab work and tests like those at Cyrex and Enterolab are so important. They help me peel back the layers and see what's going on within a patient's body. The cause of chronic pain is often overlooked, and instead of finding the root cause(s), traditional physicians prescribe painkillers or other medications that treat the symptoms rather than fixing the real problem.

THE SEVEN KEYS

1. Oxygen
    One of the big three elements the nervous system needs to function at its peak level, oxygen is necessary and essential for life. Anoxia (which means "without oxygen") equals death. Oxygen is the deal-breaker when it comes to neurological health. The less oxygen we have in our bodies, the more things start to malfunction and the less capacity our bodies have to heal themselves.
2. Glucose
    Second of the big three elements, glucose is your blood sugar. It's the fuel that your body needs to heal itself. It's also needed for the nervous system to self-regulate and function optimally. A good metaphor is that it's like

the gasoline for your car engine. Cars run at a certain octane level, and if that level gets out of balance, the car isn't going to run properly. If our blood sugar is too "low in octane" or too "high in octane," it can't function at its optimal level.

3. Stimulation

Third of the big three, stimulation's importance can't be overstated. As Einstein once said, "Nothing happens until something moves," and in the body, no healing happens until something is stimulated. Without stimulation, the body's systems weaken and fail. With proper stimulation, those systems thrive and remain strong, which is called neuroplasticity.

Oxygen > Glucose > Stimulation = Neuroplasticity

4. Autoimmune Disorders

Autoimmune disorders are kind of like "friendly fire." They develop when our immune system starts attacking the body instead of a foreign invader. Our immune system should only kill the "bad guys" like viruses and bacteria, but when it begins malfunctioning, it doesn't just destroy antigens, it also attacks our own tissues.

5. Chronic Inflammation

Logic tells you that if your house is on fire, you don't start rebuilding it until after the blazes are put out. Well, inflammation is like a fire in your body, and it can't start to heal until that fire is gone. True healing cannot take place until your body's inflammation is reduced.

6. Neurotoxins

Neurotoxins are anything that's taken into the body that causes neurological damage. Unfortunately, neurotoxins are much more common than you may imagine. Table sugar is a neurotoxin. High fructose corn syrup is a neurotoxin. The artificial sweetener Aspartame is a neurotoxin. Drinking water out of a disposable plastic bottle is neurotoxic. We'll talk more in upcoming chapters about how to eliminate these harmful toxins from your life.

7. Gut Health

    It's very simple, 70 percent of your immune system is in your gut. The role of gut health can't be overstated because poor gut health is a trigger for autoimmune conditions and out-of-control inflammatory responses. We must heal our guts to heal our brains and bodies. If you have a bad brain, you're guaranteed to have a bad gut. If you have a bad gut, you will have a bad brain. It works both ways. We must restore optimal gut health and reconnect the gut-brain axis to achieve true healing.

While each of these seven areas is important to address individually, their true power for healing comes alive when we realize that all of these elements are interconnected. Gut health and autoimmune conditions are connected. Neurotoxins and inflammation are linked. Oxygen and stimulation are crucial to one another's roles. The body is a holistic system that must be in homeostasis to heal itself and function optimally. By keeping these seven primary keys in focus, your health can transform from symptom mitigation to a state of true healing and regeneration.

CHAPTER FIVE

THE VAGUS NERVE

The secret of change is to focus all your energy, not on fighting the old, but on building the new.

—Socrates

THE VAGUS NERVE

We've touched on the vagus nerve in previous chapters, but this incredible "highway to health" easily deserves its own chapter. In the next few pages, we're diving deeply into the purpose and function of the vagus nerve, its relation to our overall health, and a few simple ways we can support this superhighway of communication through positive daily habits. By the conclusion of this chapter, you'll be a vagus nerve aficionado.

Let's begin by defining what the vagus nerve is and what it does. It is one of twelve pairs of cranial nerves, and each of these nerve pairs controls a specific area of the body. Cranial nerve number one deals with smell. Number two deals with vision. Number three controls eye movements and constricts our pupils. Numbers four and six also move our eyes. Number five deals with chewing and sensory functions of our face. Number seven controls the muscles of our facial expressions and salivation. Number eight deals with hearing and balance.

Number nine controls salivation. Number ten (the vagus nerve) deals with sensation at the back of the throat, heart rate, breathing, and digestion. Number eleven controls the trapezius muscles, and number twelve controls our tongue.

Here are a few more fun facts about the star of this chapter, the vagus nerve. The Latin word "vagus" literally translates as "wandering." The words "vagrant," "vague," and "vagabond" come from the same root. It's the longest cranial nerve in the body, which is likely how it earned its nickname "the wanderer." Our autonomic nervous system is made up of two parts: the sympathetic and parasympathetic nervous systems. The sympathetic nervous system activates the fight-or-flight response during a threat or perceived danger, and the parasympathetic nervous system restores the body to a state of calm. Cranial nerves three, seven, nine, and ten are all part of our parasympathetic nervous system (aka our "rest and digest" system).

Our sympathetic and parasympathetic nervous systems should be in homeostasis to work optimally. If we're under stress and our sympathetic nervous system gets activated, we're no longer in a rest-and-digest state; we're in a fight-or-flight mode. When we're in this state, salivation and digestion slow down because our body thinks, "Hey if the threat catches me, it doesn't matter if my food is digested or not." These are natural, God-given neurological responses designed for equipping us in immediate, stressful situations. This response should be quick and then dissipate. Unfortunately, in today's society, we're under constant stress, and this sympathetic system is ramped up all the time. The parasympathetic system isn't coming back online, so we're not resting and digesting as we should be.

How does all this chronic stress affect our friend the vagus nerve? Part of its role is maintaining optimal heart rate, breathing, and digestion. When we're under chronic stress, the vagus nerve cannot properly do its job, leading to an increased heart rate or rising blood pressure. Consequently, we begin breathing too rapidly which leads to a build-up of carbon dioxide in our body. If that happens, we can't properly rid our bodies of toxic waste. The vagus nerve is also critical in healthy gut function and controls nearly every step of our digestive process.

Let's walk through the steps of digestion so we can better understand how this system works.

When we take in food and chew it up, that's a voluntary function, but after we swallow, every step of digestion is involuntary, meaning we don't make it happen through conscious thought. As we swallow, the vagus nerve controls our upper esophageal sphincter, basically a value near the top of our esophagus that makes sure food and liquids go down the right pipe. If this sphincter isn't functioning properly, we swallow air into our stomach, which causes bloating, belching, or gas. Another sign that your valve may be leaky is if you're regularly getting food and liquids down your windpipe. This happens occasionally to everyone, but if it's happening often, it's a symptom that should be noted.

The next step of digestion is the food passing through the lower esophageal sphincter. It's also controlled by the vagus nerve, and if your vagus nerve is not functioning optimally, this sphincter may not close all the way. We have an acidic stomach which should have a pH level of 1.5–2.5 when digesting our food. If our lower esophageal sphincter isn't closing all the way, this stomach acid can back up into our esophagus.

Next, the food enters our stomach. When this happens, the vagus nerve triggers the release of hydrochloric acid (HCL), which breaks down our food into a liquid called "chime." HCL plays an important role in breaking down food, but its presence also triggers a domino effect, cueing several other important steps of digestion. While it's breaking down food in our stomach, it's also designed to kill bacteria, viruses, and parasites that may be in or on our food.

Age and the Production of HCL:

Nearly every one of my patients over the age of sixty doesn't naturally produce enough HCL to support proper digestion. To counteract this aging effect, I suggest using an HCL supplement from Apex Energetics called Enzy-mixPro (K-99). This formula combines a broad spectrum of enzymes to help support the digestion of sugars, starches, fibers, proteins, and fats. It also includes HCl for further digestive support.

If we have problems with our vagus nerve, we'll potentially have issues swallowing, experience gastric reflux, or produce an insufficient amount of HCL to digest protein or kill the bad bugs on our food. The vagus nerve controls all of the functions of our stomach, gallbladder, liver, pancreas, small intestine, and two-thirds of the large intestine. This lengthy "wanderer" controls everything from the "hangy-downy thing" at the back of your throat (uvula) to the upper portion of your colon. Physically, it travels from the back of your throat almost to your belly button.

For successful digestion to happen, every step of the process must be on point, cueing the next function in perfect rhythm just like a row of dominos. For this whole system to work in harmony, the vagus nerve serves as the superhighway of communication between the brain and the digestive system. Every part of the digestive system sends messages back to the brain saying, "Hey, this is what we're doing down here." If these organs start going rogue and acting of their own accord, they get out of sync, malfunction, and food products can't be assimilated properly, which sets up the perfect conditions for a disease process to take root.

The most amazing fact about the vagus nerve is that only 20 percent of its job is sending signals from the brain to the gut. The remaining 80 percent of its function is sending messages up to the brain from the gut. For example, once food reaches the stomach, the stomach sends a message back to the brain saying, "Hey, I'm releasing the right amount of HCL."

The gallbladder says, "Yep, I'm secreting bile."

The small intestine says, "Yes, my tight junctions are closed off so bad stuff doesn't get into the bloodstream."

The large intestine says, "Yep, I'm doing my job and removing water from the stool."

Then the microbiome says, "Yep, I'm assisting in the regulation of the immune system."

All of those messages are sent up through the vagus nerve to the brain to let it know everything is under control down below. Even more amazing is that all of this is happening without our conscious thought. Our conscious mind is completely unaware of this activity until we've damaged enough tissue that we're having pain, bloating, distension, constipation, diarrhea, or gastric reflex. That's when symptoms show up.

Envision digestion as a road trip. The journey has a set route getting you from point A to point B. If the car runs well, you have enough fuel, and you read your map correctly, the road trip goes smoothly and you reach your destination without a problem. However, if you have a flat tire, run out of gas, or miss your turn, the trip becomes complicated in a hurry. Digestion is the same way. If something breaks down from the point where we swallow our food until it reaches our colon, we get symptoms that may lead to disease processes. So, what are the first signs of breakdown? Gastric reflux, bloating, distension, diarrhea, excessive gas, and constipation are some initial signs of dysfunction. If they aren't addressed, these early symptoms progress into disease processes such as inflammatory bowel syndrome (IBS), gastroesophageal reflux disease (GERD), and small intestinal bacterial overgrowth (SIBO).

You may be surprised to hear that conditions like multiple sclerosis (MS), Parkinson's disease, fibromyalgia, ADD, ADHD, and dyslexia are also hugely related to gut function. Nearly every neurological disease starts in the gut before manifesting in the brain, and all of these conditions, if caught early enough, may be helped. The most effective way of healing the body is by addressing all three areas, brain, body, and gut, at the same time. We can make progress by treating the gut exclusively, the brain exclusively, or the vagus nerve exclusively, but true transformation happens when all three are treated simultaneously.

THE NERVE IN ACTION

Think of the vagus nerve as a telephone wire. The brain is on one end of the conversation and the gut is on the other. The vagus nerve is the phone wire enabling communication between the two parties. When the phone system is working well, they speak clearly, quickly, and efficiently, allowing both parties to get their messages across. When the phone line is garbled or has a dead spot, the messages get mixed up. Imagine your spouse calling and asking you to pick up some chicken for dinner. They clearly say "chicken," but just as the words come out of their mouth, you hit a dead spot, and it sounds like "broccoli" instead. You happily pick up broccoli from the store and head home, excitedly giving your spouse their requested ingredient, but alas, it was the wrong thing and dinner is ruined. Communication is important.

In the same way, a healthy vagus nerve ensures clear communication between the brain and gut. An unhealthy vagus nerve isn't just a dead spot of thirty to forty-five seconds, it's a 24/7 malfunction that doesn't correct itself until you see a professional who can diagnose the problem and help you get the system back online.

You may be wondering, "If keeping the vagus nerve healthy is this important, what can I do in my daily life to support it?" Excellent question. Before we get into supporting it, let's talk about what to stop doing. Here are three things you may be doing in your daily life that are unconsciously harming your vagus nerve:

1. Getting on social media (e.g., Facebook, Instagram) or turning on the news first thing in the morning, creating chronic stress. Right out of the gate, this hits your nervous system with bad news, negative thought processes, and comparisons. That inundation with bad news leads to stress. That constant stress causes an imbalance between the sympathetic and parasympathetic nervous systems, which raises our heart rate, slows down digestion, and causes a cascade of other dysfunctions.

2. Eating a SAD. The standard American's morning looks something like this: wake up, gripe and complain about going to work, eat a sugary, carb-laden breakfast (e.g., pastry, pancakes, sugary cereal) chock full of gluten, hydrogenated oils, and other preservatives, then turn on the news or get on the internet and be inundated with stress. In this morning routine, the body is hit with physical stress (bad diet) and psychological stress (complaining, negative attitude, and bad news). The body doesn't differentiate between those two forms of stress that put an extra load on the vagus nerve, and the inflammatory processes triggered by these foods can damage our brains, nerve function, and gut function.

3. Living a sedentary lifestyle. A sedentary lifestyle is directly hurting your vagus nerve by not stimulating your brain through exercise, and thus not stimulating your vagus nerve. Studies have shown a direct correlation between muscles getting smaller and your brain actually shrinking. Movement is vital to brain health, and brain health is vital to gut health because of the vagus nerve connecting them.

Three things I can do to support my vagus nerve:

1. Exercise: The simplest way to do this is by walking. When you stimulate the body through exercise, you also stimulate the brain, which stimulates the vagus nerve. This has wonderful effects on your gut-brain connection. Make a commitment to move at least four days per week for twenty minutes per day.

2. Deep breathing exercises: This is an ultra-simple way of supporting the vagus nerve. At least once per day,

intentionally focus on inhaling for eight seconds, then exhaling for sixteen seconds, ten times in a row. This rush of oxygen stimulates the brain and supports the vagus nerve's function.

3. Ice bath or cold shower: Ice baths or cold showers stimulate our sympathetic and parasympathetic nervous systems, decrease our stress response, improve our immune system, aid in weight loss, and improve tissue recovery processes, all of which contribute to a natural high, boosting mood and attitude. I take forty-eight to fifty-three degree ice baths four days per week for fifteen minutes at a time. A simple way to start this habit is by incorporating it into your daily shower. Take your normal, warm shower, then turn on the cold water for one minute at the end. Once you're regularly doing this, progress to having the warm water on for two minutes, then cold water for one minute, and do that for three cycles. Note: Please speak to your doctor before starting ice baths.

Bonus: You can access vagus nerve therapy exercises in my first book, *License to Heal*. For additional vagus nerve therapies and exercises, check out pages 93–94.

All of these exercises and habits are grounded in commitment. We all have an expiration date, and we must take action today and every day to ensure our bodies are as healthy as possible. Next let's dig into the ABCs to Health that will give you an initial road map to follow.

CHAPTER SIX

THE ABCs TO HEALTH

I believe that the only courage anybody ever needs is the courage to follow your own dream.

—Oprah Winfrey

ABCs TO HEATH

This is one of my favorite chapters because what follows is a simple recipe for drastically improved health: the ABCs TO HEALTH. If you follow these steps, your life and health will be revitalized. Your inflammation will decrease, your body function will increase, and your brain (and vagus nerve) function will increase as well. All of these wonderful benefits come from making small but important lifestyle improvements. Chronic diseases are also known as "lifestyle diseases" because it's often our daily habits and lifestyle that create them over time. In the same way, we can change our habits using the ABCs to Health as our guide and reverse many of the symptoms of chronic disease.

This book is all about the gut-brain-body connection so before we define the ABCs TO HEALTH, let's discuss why they matter to this vital superhighway of communication in our bodies.

1. By following the ABCs TO HEALTH, your overall inflammation will decrease, which lessens the strain on your brain, vagus nerve, and gut and allows your body to heal itself.

2. Your brain health and function will improve, which also supercharges your healing journey.

3. The overall health of your microbiome will improve.

What is your microbiome, you ask? The human microbiome consists of 100 trillion symbiotic microbial cells, primarily bacteria, located in our guts. There are ten times more bacteria, fungi, and viruses in the gut microbiome than cells in our body, and it weighs about three pounds, which is similar to the weight of a human brain. Nevertheless, the gut microbiome has long been forgotten. Only within the last five to ten years has the world of scientific research homed in on understanding this amazing ecosystem inside of us. Rest assured, by following the ABCs TO HEALTH, your gut microbiome will soon be thriving.

Let's dive into this quick action guide for fast-tracking your health. Just as you follow a recipe to bake a cake or make cookies (gluten free, of course), this is the recipe for optimizing your health. If you follow this recipe, good things *will* happen.

ABCs TO HEALTH: THE ACRONYM

A. Antioxidants

Why They Matter: Antioxidants are our body's defense against free radicals, a type of unstable molecule made during cellular metabolism (the set of chemical reactions that occur in living organisms to maintain life), that can build up in cells and cause a state known as oxidative stress. This may damage your DNA and other important structures in your cells, and this damage can increase the risk of cancer and other diseases. Although free radicals are produced naturally in the body, lifestyle factors such as trauma, stress, poor diet, or living a sedentary lifestyle can accelerate their production.

Imagine a boxing match where in one corner we have the free radicals, and in the other corner are the antioxidants. Free radicals are the bad guys and antioxidants are the good guys. The bell dings, and the free radicals and antioxidants duke it out. Antioxidants defeat the free radicals by neutralizing them which decreases overall inflammation in the body. Basically, increasing antioxidants means decreasing the harmful effects of free radicals.

Today's Action Step: Increase your consumption of antioxidants by eating more carrots, broccoli, asparagus, berries, artichokes, kale, cabbage, and beets. The natural color of a food is a great indicator of its antioxidant content so make your plate as colorful as naturally possible.

The Next Level: Take a daily supplement from Apex Energetics called ADEK Pro (K102), which contains powerful amounts of antioxidants.

B. Brain-Based Therapy
Why It Matters: It's always the right time to take care of your noggin. We need a healthy brain to function in society, and it's also crucial to digestion and gut health because it's the start of the vagus nerve.

Today's Action Step: Get off the couch and get walking. This is the easiest, fastest way of activating and stimulating your brain function, and since stimulation is one of the seven keys to health, the brain must be stimulated to maintain optimal function.

The Next Level: Schedule an appointment for a Clear Mind brain map. This is a computerized system that takes a functional image of your brain. It tells us not only which lobes of the brain are weak and need help but also shows in detail which lobes of the brain are healthy and functioning properly. The procedure takes about forty minutes.

C. Clean Gut and Clean Brain

Why It Matters: In the last few decades, poor nutritional habits, stressful lifestyles, and chemical exposures have created significant health problems for our society. We can fight these environmental factors by supporting two of the body's key functions: digestion and detoxification. Detoxing (cleaning out) the brain and the gut simultaneously multiplies the positive effects of detoxification and removes the toxin load hampering our body from doing its number one job, healing itself.

The body's accumulated toxins are embedded in different tissues like fat and connective tissues. Before removing these toxins from the body, they first must be mobilized aka "released" from the areas where they're hiding. After they're mobilized, they enter the detoxification pathways, and after the detoxification reactions, the leftover compounds are excreted from the body.

Today's Action Step: Start supporting your body's digestion and detoxification using something you likely have in your pantry, apple cider vinegar. Make sure it's an unrefined vinegar containing the "mother," which is the healthy, good-for-you bacteria formed during the fermentation of the vinegar. Combine thirty-three ounces of water with two ounces of apple cider vinegar and drink it throughout the day.

The Next Level: Commit to doing Apex Energetics' "Repair & Clear™ Program" a ten-week system specifically designed for powerful detoxification and digestive support.

S.   Stop the SAD Diet and SAL Lifestyle

Why It Matters: As we've discussed in earlier chapters, the SAD is devastating to our health. It is chock full of gluten, unhealthy fats, sugar, excessively starchy carbohydrates, and other inflammation-causing foods. There's zero chance of reclaiming health and vitality if we continue eating this way, and the Standard American Lifestyle (SAL) isn't any better. It's sedentary, lacks physical stimulation and exercise, and relies on hours of TV or other screen time for numbing the negative emotional, physical, and mental side effects it causes. SAD and SAL must go if restoring our health and promoting our bodies' abilities to heal themselves is our goal.

Today's Action Step: Stop eating gluten and processed foods because we can't start getting better until we stop making it worse. Commit to walking (preferably outdoors) for 20 minutes per day, four times per week.

The Next Level: Eat fruits, vegetables, salads, raw nuts (almonds, walnuts, pecans), organic meats (bison, beef, chicken, fish, wild game).

T. Time Out, Relax, and Reset

Why It Matters: Taking a moment for quiet reflection and relaxation gives your brain the time it needs for a "reset." Stress is one of the leading causes of inflammation, leaky gut, depression, anxiety, and insomnia. Focusing on deep breathing and meditation encourages your brain to return to a rest-and-digest state, letting your body know it doesn't need to worry about fight-or-flight anymore.

Today's Action Step: Sit in a quiet room and do focused deep breathing exercises for ten minutes. Turn your phone off. Focus on positive things rather than negative things. Think about a loved one or a vacation you want to take. Listen to nature sounds.

The Next Level: Create a daily habit of meditation and focused breathing. Bonus points for doing it twice per day. Get a massage once a month. You deserve it.

O. Omega 3 Fish Oil

Why It Matters: Omega 3 fish oil is a wonderful health supplement for restoring brain and nerve function. Seventy-five percent of the weight of our brain is fat, and the myelin sheath (coating around our nerves) is also made of fat. Fatty fish is a rich source of Omega-3 fatty acids, a major building block of the brain. Omega-3s play a role in sharpening memory and improving mood, as well as protecting your brain against cognitive decline.

Today's Action Step: Take a high-quality Omega 3 supplement every day. If you've had bad experiences with fish oil supplements, you probably weren't taking a high-quality version, or you may have gallbladder issues.

The Next Level: Take a high-quality Omega 3 supplement every day and eat fatty fish like salmon, mackerel, tuna, herring, and sardines two to three times per week. Nuts and seeds like flaxseed, chia seeds, and walnuts are great sources of Omega 3 as well.

H. High-Fiber Diet
    Why It Matters: Eating a high fiber diet helps regulate the body's use of sugars, helping to keep hunger and blood sugar in check. Fiber also supports regular bowel movements and consistent digestion.

    Today's Action Step: The old saying goes, "An apple a day keeps the doctor away," and it's still true. Eat real fruits and vegetables, not fruit juice. Aim to eat one fruit per day and at least one green, leafy vegetable per day.

    The Next Level: Drink a daily smoothie containing protein, fat, fiber, and greens. Excellent sources of fiber include chia seeds, whole fruits, and vegetables.

E. Exercise with Oxygen Therapy (EWOT)
    Why It Matters: Forced breathing exercises activate your frontal lobe and increase the oxygen supply in the body. Oxygen is needed to optimize brain and body function.

    Today's Action Step: Keep your brain and body strong by walking for at least twenty minutes per day, four times per week. While walking, do forced breathing exercises to supercharge your brain's oxygen supply.

    The Next Level: Supplement with nitric balance (K-62) from Apex Energetics. It helps dilate blood vessels for improved circulation, mental clarity, and body performance.

A. Avoid Gluten and Casein

Why It Matters: Avoid gluten and casein (the protein in dairy) at all costs as they can lead to inflammation, leaky gut, and many other chronic diseases.

Today's Action Step: Remove gluten and dairy from your diet and take GlutenFlam (K52) from Apex Energetics anytime you eat out or may be exposed to cross-contamination of gluten or casein.

The Next Level: Take the Enterolab A2 test, a panel that tests for sensitivity to the four primary individual food antigens (gluten, milk, eggs, and soy) and includes a gene test for understanding your genetic predisposition to gluten sensitivity and celiac disease.

L. Lactobacillus and Bifidobacterium (Take a high-quality probiotic.)

Why It Matters: Probiotics help heal the gut, support your microbiome, unlock optimal digestion, boost weight loss, support your immune system, and promote overall health.

Today's Action Step: Start taking a high quality probiotic every day I use and recommend Strengtia (K-61) from Apex Energetics, but there are several great ones on the market. Make sure your probiotic of choice supplies at least 10 billion colony-forming units. If they're lower than that, they're not worth your money.

The Next Level: In addition to your daily probiotic supplement, make fermented foods like plain dairy-free yogurt (Silk yogurt made from almonds or SO Delicious yogurt made from coconut milk), traditionally prepared sauerkraut, kombucha, kimchi, or traditionally made pickles a regular part of your diet.

T. Time to Heal

Why It Matters: Have you ever built or remodeled a home? It always takes 40–50 percent longer than you expect. Healing the body is the same way. It didn't become dysfunctional overnight, and it's not going to heal overnight. It needs plenty of time, rest, and support to fully heal itself.

Today's Action Step: Commit to giving your body ample time to heal. Resist rushing the process or giving unrealistic expectations a foothold.

The Next Level: Write out the ultimate life you envision then go back and review this vision statement whenever you're feeling discouraged or rushed in your health journey.

H. Hydrochloric Acid (HCL)

Why It Matters: When digesting food, your stomach acid should have a pH level of 1.5–2.5. When the level of acidity is off in the stomach, all kinds of problems occur. First, if the stomach doesn't have enough HCL, food isn't broken down properly, and the possible viruses, bacteria, and parasites in our food aren't destroyed. Second, the next steps of digestion aren't triggered properly. The domino effect we talked about earlier doesn't take place. Almost no one over the age of sixty is producing enough HCL.

Today's Action Step: Start taking EnzymixPro (K99) from Apex Energetics. This HCL supporting supplement ensures your food is properly broken down and the next steps of digestion are triggered correctly.

The Next Level: Add apple cider vinegar to your diet and do your vagus nerve stimulation daily.

The ABCs TO HEALTH are a simple, easy-to-follow recipe to wellness. By following these steps, you're sending yourself squarely down the middle of the highway to health. They aren't complicated or expensive, but for fun, let's simplify these action steps even more. Pretend you're sitting across from me at my office and ask, "Dr. Barlow, what are the top three most important things I can start doing today to improve my health?"

This is my answer:

1) Get your HCL levels cranking. Having the right amount of acidity in the stomach is absolutely critical to setting up the rest of your gut for success. Order the Apex Energetics "K99" EnzymixPro today, and take it daily after every meal.

2) Stop eating gluten and casein today. They are detrimental to your health and devastating to your gut. Cut them out now, and start a detox program like the ten-week Brain and Body Detox from Apex Energetics.

3) Get out and get walking. Commit to walking for at least twenty minutes per day, four days a week. This form of exercise is easy, free, and takes minimal time, yet it stimulates your body, which in turn stimulates your brain and vagus nerve, increases your oxygen supply, and improves your mood.

Now that you've read the recipe to the highway to health, let's walk through the way every bite you take directly impacts your gut-brain connection.

CHAPTER SEVEN

THE TEN-STORY BUILDING IN YOUR BODY

We are all here for a reason. Stop being a prisoner of our past. Become the architect of your future.

—Robin Sharma

THE TEN STORIES

Digestion is a complex process, but it doesn't have to remain a mystery. Digestion is meant to mechanically break down food (which happens in the stomach) while absorption of food products occurs in the small intestine and is assisted by the liver, gallbladder, and pancreas. We can easily understand all the steps of digestion using the analogy of a ten-story building. You can only get from the top of the building to the bottom by going through every floor, just like digestion. Every part of the process is important and sets up the next step to complete its role.

FLOOR #10: CHEWING

Digestion runs from top to bottom and in the same way, our analogy begins on floor number ten. Imagine you've just taken a big bite of an apple. This triggers the start of the digestive process, which actually begins in your mouth. Pro tip: chew your food at least twenty times to cue the enzymes needed to kick off proper digestion. Chewing is the mechanical breakdown of food, and the "muscles of mastication" are run by cranial nerve number five.

FLOOR #9: SALIVATION

Run by cranial nerves seven and nine, salivation produces saliva that contains special enzymes that start digesting your food. An enzyme called amylase breaks down starches into sugars, and an enzyme called lingual lipase begins breaking down fats.

FLOOR #8: SWALLOWING

Swallowing involves the upper esophageal sphincter and lower esophageal sphincter, which are both controlled by the vagus nerve. From this point forward, the autonomic nervous system takes over, and we no longer have conscious thought about our digestion. When things go awry at this stage, you may experience acid reflux, which happens when the lower esophageal sphincter allows acid from the stomach back up into the esophagus. Traditional doctors usually prescribe proton pump inhibiting medications like Prilosec or Nexium for this condition. Unfortunately, these drugs cause more problems down the line because they actually change the pH level of the stomach. Studies have linked the use of proton pump inhibiting medications to an eight to nine times increase in colon cancer. Signs that your lower esophageal sphincter is malfunctioning include regularly burping forty-five to fifty minutes after eating food, getting acid reflux when lying down at night, or bloating, distension, and gas.

FLOOR #7: STOMACH

Also controlled by the vagus nerve, this is where food is further broken down by the enzyme pepsin and HCL into chyme.

FLOOR #6: GALLBLADDER

Prompted by HCL production in the stomach, the gallbladder contracts and releases bile into the small intestine, which aids in breaking down fats. If you have pain in the upper right quadrant of your torso sixty to seventy-five minutes after eating, that's a sign that your gallbladder is struggling.

FLOOR #5: SMALL INTESTINE

This is where the majority of our food is digested and absorbed. The lining of the small intestine resembles a screen door (keeps the bugs out, lets the air in), and it's what protects us from the outside world that's in our food. This lining is made of tiny tight junctions that have microvilli (think little squiggles that resemble shag carpet) coming off of them. When things are working as they should, these tight junctions are so close together that only good things can pass through (e.g., amino acids, vitamins, minerals) into the portal vein that passes through our liver and ends up in our bloodstream. When leaky gut happens, those tight junctions loosen and become leaky, allowing all kinds of bad things to pass through (e.g., undigested proteins, gluten, bacteria) that should not get through the lining of the small intestine.

FLOOR #4: LIVER

The liver's job is twofold: 1) producing bile, which it sends to the gallbladder, to break down fat for digestion and 2) filtering everything that comes from our small intestine before it reaches our bloodstream. Everything we put in our mouths is filtered through our liver.

FLOOR #3: PANCREAS

The pancreas releases crucial digestive enzymes that break down proteins, sugars, fats, and starches. Your pancreas also helps your digestive system by making hormones (insulin being one of them), which are the chemical messengers that travel through your blood. If you have pain or discomfort roughly two hours after eating protein, that could be a sign your pancreas is struggling.

FLOOR #2: COLON

There are three divisions of the colon: 1) ascending, 2) transverse, and 3) descending. The main job of the colon is to absorb water from feces before it's eliminated from the body. It's also home to our microbiome.

FLOOR #1: ELIMINATION THROUGH THE RECTUM

The final step of digestion is getting rid of the remnants by ejecting them out of the rectum.

Along this path of digestion, if we have problems with any of these "stories" or phases, we always work top down to find the origin of the dysfunction. Armed with this new knowledge, here are the action steps you can take today to make sure you're on the highway to gut and brain health.

1. METABOLIC SUPPORT

The most important thing you can do is get all the equipment working on the inside. Start caring for your gut and brain health by following the ABCs to Health (see the previous chapter) and completing a ten-week brain and body detox. Why invest in the ten-week detox? It will accomplish several important metabolic goals: 1) helps with focus and attention disorders, anxiety, insomnia, and depression by detoxing your brain and gut; 2) decreases pain and inflammation by detoxing your body; 3) helps heal the gut lining which is crucial to your long-term health because seventy percent of your immune system is in your gut; 4) probably causes a fifteen to twenty pound weight loss; and 5) helps detox the liver and pancreas.

2. LAB WORK AND METABOLIC TESTING

If you're serious about healing your body, untangling the web of dysfunction, and getting on the highway to health, these tests are game changers. I recommend the following tests to create a clear, comprehensive picture of your current health:

1. Chem 77 blood test, which analyzes glucose, inflammation, anemia, liver and kidney function;
2. Enterolab A2 panel, which detects gluten and celiac genes as well as malabsorption issues;
3. Cyrex Array #2, which is the leaky gut test; and

4. Cyrex Array #5, which reveals any kind of autoimmune disorder you have brewing or that has already
   manifested.

If you're living with chronic health problems or you
simply want to be proactive about your health and longevity,
the information revealed through these tests is crucial.

3. EXERCISE CONSISTENTLY

At the risk of sounding like a broken record, I'll say it again.
Commit to exercising for twenty minutes per day, at least
four days per week.

If you want to go "all-out" for your health and have these
tests done, call my office at 662-844-1414, and I'll either set
you up with the tests or I'll recommend a doctor in your area
who can administer them for you. I or a doctor I recommend
can also get you started on the ten-week detox program and
any other supplements you need. In the next chapter, we're
going to discuss the leaky gut, break down what causes this
condition, and look at ways we can solve this problem.

CHAPTER EIGHT

LEAKY GUT

*Success is a personal standard, reaching
for the highest that is in us, becoming
all we can be.*

—Zig Ziglar

WHAT IS LEAKY GUT?

We've touched on this greatly misunderstood condition in previous chapters, but now let's take a chapter to really define leaky gut, identify its causes, and look at methods for healing it. This often misunderstood and overlooked condition is at the heart of many chronic illnesses, and if you struggle with a chronic disease, it may be one of the root causes of your web of dysfunction.

As in the ten-story building analogy, leaky gut appears in the small intestine. The number one way to test for this condition is the Cyrex Array #2 test. There are many signs and symptoms that can point to this diagnosis, but the only way to be sure is by doing this test. Leaky gut develops in the lining of the small intestine. Discovered in 2000 by Alessio Fasano and his team at the University of Maryland School of Medicine, this lining consists of tight junctions (aka the screen door) and microvilli (aka the shag carpet). The tight junctions look and act like a screen door, keeping the bad guys (bugs) out and allowing the good guys to pass through (a cool summer's breeze). When the lining of the small intestine is healthy, only amino acids (digested proteins that are the building blocks of life) and nutrients pass through this lining. Trouble arises when the tight junctures of an unhealthy gut lining loosen and allow undigested proteins to pass through, causing inflammation throughout the body. Think of the neighborhood kid throwing a baseball through the screen door of your house. Once the screen door is breached, bugs can get in your home and spread quickly.

Since the path from the small intestine to the blood-stream is the small intestine > portal vein > liver > blood stream, the liver is the body's first line of defense against these invaders. Once the bad guys get past the liver, they go into our bloodstream, traveling to every corner of our bodies and becoming a systemic problem. They tend to settle into whichever system of the body is the weakest link, which is why the symptoms of leaky gut can be vastly different from one person to the next. One person may suffer from frontal lobe issues like depression and focus and attention issues, whereas the next deals with parietal lobe problems of chronic pain, fibromyalgia. Still others experience gut issues such as gastric reflux, bloating, and constipation or numbness and tingling in the hands and feet. Each of these individuals is seeing every doctor under the sun, taking their meds, and continuing to suffer, and yet my patients tell me they've never heard the words "leaky gut" until they came to my office.

The body knows these undigested proteins shouldn't be traveling freely throughout the bloodstream, so it tries eliminating them from the body using one of the five organs of elimination: liver, lungs, skin, kidneys, and colon. Interestingly, rates of cancer in all of these organs of elimination are skyrocketing. Could it be that our systems are overworked, overstressed, and maxed out to the point that our God-given methods of elimination can't keep up? The rates of disease in these organs certainly point in that direction.

When a person's gut is leaky, they may experience symptoms in a variety of ways. Even though your root issue is a leaky gut, your greatest symptom may not be gut-related at all. It could be settling and manifesting elsewhere in the body. Here are the main three areas I see leaky gut symptoms appear in my patients:

1. In the body, symptoms appear as joint pain, fibromyalgia, or undiagnosed chronic pain.
2. In the brain, symptoms manifest as anxiety, depression, insomnia, focus and attention issues, or other neurodegenerative conditions.
3. In the gut, symptoms show up as IBS, gluten sensitivity or celiac disease, constipation, diarrhea, and bloating.

The effects of leaky gut should be thought of from two perspectives: short-term and long term. They show up in three main areas: the brain, body, and gut. In the brain, the short-term impact of leaky gut shows up as insomnia, depression, anxiety, and focus and concentration problems. If left untreated, the possible long-term effects can grow into serious diseases like Alzheimer's, dementia, and Parkinson's.

The short-term impact of leaky gut in the body can appear as joint pain, slight tingling in hands and feet, or fibromyalgia. Again, when left untreated, these less obvious symptoms progress into major obstacles like mobility and balance problems, needing the help of a cane or walker, and severe neuropathy. When looking at the gut, short-term effects of leaky gut appear as gas, stomach pain, bloating, distension, diarrhea, or constipation. In the long-term, these seemingly "normal" digestive issues grow into bigger problems like IBS, Crohn's, and other severe digestive illnesses. Leaky gut is a serious condition that should be treated with urgency and commitment. One of the biggest misconceptions in the medical world today is that leaky gut is a figment of holistic doctors' imaginations, not the root cause of chronic disease for millions of people around the world.

There's perhaps no area of disease where this is more misunderstood than in neurological disorders. Brain degeneration, such as Alzheimer's, typically happens in seven stages, and when you know the seven stages, you're able to pinpoint where you or your loved ones may be on the spectrum.

BRAIN DEGENERATION DOMINO EFFECT: (SEVEN STAGES OF ALZHEIMER'S)

Stage 1: Normal outward behavior.

Stage 2: Very mild cognitive changes and mental fatigue. I've seen this in patients as early as thirty years of age.

Stage 3: Mild decline. Focus, attention, and concentration issues and/or brain fog. Again, I have seen this in patients as early as thirty years of age.

Stage 4: Moderate decline. Working memory issues. Getting lost in conversation. You walk in a room and forget why you walked in the room. You can't remember where you parked your car at the mall. Usually I see this in patients in their fifth or sixth decade of life. You, your family, and even your doctor shrug it off, saying, "You're getting older, you know." Give me a break. This is not normal. It's common, but not normal.

Stage 5: Moderate to severe decline. You lose your keys, phone, remote, or coffee cup. You think others are playing tricks on you because you keep losing things. You get lost while driving. You start blaming others for all your problems.

Stage 6: Severe decline. You can't remember the name of your spouse or children. It is a very sad situation for everyone involved.

Stage 7: End stage. Unable to walk and requires significant assistance with ambulation. This stage lasts an average of 2.5 years.

Here's the point: if you are waiting for a dementia or Alzheimer's diagnosis, it probably won't happen until the fifth or sixth stage, and by then it's too late. Think of all the years and decades wasted where you could've been treating the root cause. Leaky gut is not a condition to be taken lightly. Even though the brain, body, and gut symptoms may start out mild, if left unchecked, this condition will tarnish your quality of life and create a web of health dysfunction.

With all of this talk about why we should take leaky gut seriously, it's natural to ask, "Well, where does it come from?"

Here are the three leading causes of leaky gut:

1. Prior head trauma. This could be from a car wreck twenty years ago or a sports injury in high school. Studies have shown that within six hours of head trauma, you may develop a leaky brain and a leaky gut because of the stress and shock to the brain and vagus nerve. Very few doctors will ever ask you about your past head trauma if you see them for gastrointestinal issues or brain-based symptoms, yet the science is clear: brain trauma decreases firing of the brain > decreases firing of the vagus nerve > decreases activation of tight junctions

in the small intestine > creates leaky gut > bad bugs flow through portal vein > reach and pass through liver > systemic inflammation.

2. Glucose dysregulation. This issue leads to inflammation in the brain, gut, and body, causing the brain to slow down. When the brain slows down, this domino effect occurs: brain activity decreases > vagus nerve can't maintain the integrity of the tight junctions in small intestine > creates leaky gut > bad bugs get through portal vein to liver > systemic inflammation.

3. Gluten sensitivity. This leads to systemic inflammation and potential autoimmunity to brain, gut, and body tissues. Talk about a double whammy. Again, this leads to slowing down the brain > decreased function of the vagus nerve > inability to maintain tight junctions > leaky gut > portal vein > systemic inflammation.

LEAKY GUT SOLUTIONS

Healing a leaky gut is a process requiring time, consistency, and commitment. Like all chronic health problems, it didn't become dysfunctional overnight, and it's not going to heal overnight either. However, you can get on the highway to health by healing your leaky gut and supporting your gut-brain connection through the following actions:

1) Stop eating processed foods, dairy, and gluten.
2) Increase your fiber and nutrient intake by eating more natural, colorful fruits and vegetables.
3) Add high-quality probiotics and naturally prepared fermented foods to your daily diet.

4) Bonus Action Item: Take your healing to the next level by committing to a ten-week Clearvite and RepairVite Brain and Body Detox.

When you take these daily steps to change your habits and heal your leaky gut, you'll notice several results. First, if your gut is in the condition of most Americans, you'll experience a seven- to ten-day detox period. Why does this happen? Because changing your diet and eating clean essentially starves all the bad bugs in your gut, and when they starve, they begin to die. As they die off, they release waste products and toxins. This "die-off" effect may create unpleasant cramping, diarrhea, and sometimes constipation. Typically the more intense your detox phase, the more toxic your gut was in the beginning. The great news is that once your gut is cleaned out, you immediately begin reaping the rewards of your hard work and commitment. Your focus, attention, concentration, and ability to sleep soundly will improve. Your chronic aches and pains will lessen. Your attitude will likely improve, and you may lose weight. Your overall inflammation will decrease immensely, and your energy should skyrocket.

Making these lifestyle changes shouldn't be painful or miserable. Like any new habit, there will be an adjustment period. It'll take two weeks for your taste buds to adjust to your new way of eating, and you'll have to learn new ways of satisfying those sweet treat cravings, but you can do it. Instead of eating a candy bar, grab an apple. Rather than eating a slice of pie for dessert, enjoy some dairy-free yogurt topped with fresh-cut fruit. Give yourself time and grace as you learn a new way of living and eating. I promise the results you'll feel will be worth every sacrifice. Now that we've covered leaky gut and its relationship to autoimmune disorders, let's move to the next key to solving chronic health problems: controlling stomach acid.

CHAPTER NINE

WHEN FOOD BECOMES YOUR ENEMY

It is never too late to be the person you might have been.

—George Eliot

WHAT IS HYPOCHLORHYDRIA?

This all-to-common condition happens when the stomach doesn't produce enough hydrochloric acid (HCL). When we're digesting food, the pH balance (level of acidity) of the stomach should be between 1.5 and 2.5. The scale of acidity ranges from zero to fourteen with zero being the absolute most acidic and fourteen being the most alkaline, or basic. When the pH level of the stomach becomes too basic, problems arise because there's not enough acid in the stomach to properly digest food. When the stomach isn't acidic enough, a cascade of negative effects occur.

First, our food isn't totally broken down, allowing undigested proteins to pass through into the small intestine. This stresses the lining of the small intestine and sets the stage for leaky gut. It also means our bodies can't break down our food products into vitamins and minerals. Second, the proper amount of HCL is needed to kill the bad bugs, parasites, and viruses that come into our systems in and on our food. Third, a shortage of HCL means other important steps of digestion which should be cued by HCL aren't activated. Steps like prompting the gallbladder to release bile or the pancreas to release essential digestive enzymes are missed because there's not enough HCL to trigger the action. The fourth negative side effect of too little HCL is a bit counterintuitive. Acid reflux is thought to happen when you have too much stomach acid, but the opposite is actually true. Most often, acid reflux is a result of too little stomach acid also known as hypochlorhydria.

When hypochlorhydria is reversed, you'll notice the following positive effects:

1) Diminished bloating, gas, and belching.

2) Protein is properly broken down into essential amino acids, the molecules that are the right size to easily pass through the lining of the small intestine. If you're curious how the breakdown of protein relates to battling depression, one of the amino acids needed to produce serotonin (the "happy" hormone that stabilizes mood and nurtures feelings of well-being) is tryptophan. If your body can't break protein down into tryptophan, it can't produce enough serotonin, which leads to anxiety and depression symptoms.

3) Your body correctly breaks down essential vitamins and minerals providing relief from malabsorption syndrome.

4) The proper amount of HCL in the stomach relieves IBS, spurs the gallbladder to work properly, and prompts the pancreas to release digestive enzymes to break down fats, proteins, and carbs.

As you can see, having the right level and amount of stomach acid is important for every stage of digestion. The good news is that we can reverse hypochlorhydria with a few simple lifestyle and diet adjustments. When we get the fundamentals of digestion right, we can sit back and let the body heal. Think of optimizing your digestion as pouring the foundation of a home. Nothing else in the home can be square, sturdy, and long lasting unless the foundation is laid correctly.

The tell-tale symptoms of hypochlorhydria are:

1. Heartburn and acid reflux. This condition is actually a symptom of an environment that's not acidic enough. For example, a reduced amount of stomach acid can lead to an increase of intra-abdominal pressure (IAP), which can cause the lower esophageal sphincter to open, allowing small amounts of stomach acid to touch the esophagus and cause the familiar burning sensation experienced in gastric reflux.

2. Gallbladder discomfort. If you feel discomfort on the right side of your torso, under your rib cage, about an hour after eating, this can be a sign that your gallbladder is sluggish. Your gallbladder becomes sluggish when it's not contracting properly and releasing bile to help break down fats. This happens when there's not enough HCL to trigger the gallbladder to contract as it should.

3. Pancreas pain. If you feel pain in your upper abdomen about two hours after eating, this can be a sign your pancreas isn't producing or releasing enough digestive enzymes to break down protein and starchy foods. If your pancreas isn't producing enough enzymes, you may also notice flatulence or diarrhea after eating green, leafy vegetables.

Why does this happen? What causes someone's stomach to lack HCL? The first and most mysterious cause of hypochlorhydria is past trauma to the brain. The vagus nerve has to stimulate and activate the stomach to kick off digestion. Head trauma from many years previous can damage the brain and/or vagus nerve, slowing down communication between the brain and the gut. This dysfunction takes months or years to build up, so most people (and their doctors) don't correlate it with the digestive problems they're having today. Car wrecks, football injuries, soccer collisions, falling off a horse, a cheerleading injury, a four-wheeler wreck: the list goes on. All of these head injuries contribute to chronic health issues later in life.

The next reason hypochlorhydria develops is a rogue bacteria called *H. pylori*. This bad actor is present in the guts of 50–75 percent of the world's population, and for many, it doesn't cause a problem. Unfortunately, it can get into the stomach and wreak havoc on your health and HCL production. If it grows out of control, it drastically alters your stomach and gut function. If you have stomach or duodenal ulcers, definitely ask your doctor about being tested for *H. pylori*. The third and most common reason people don't produce enough HCL is age. Production of hydrochloric acid goes down drastically after the age of sixty.

HYPOCHLORHYDRIA SOLUTIONS

Now let's talk about methods of fixing the problem so you can get back to living your best life. The first and most important thing to rule out is an *H. pylori* infection. *H. pylori* overgrowth is serious and can lead to ulcers in your stomach. The most common treatment for *H. pylori* is antibiotics. There is a time and a place for prescription drugs, and this is one of those times. There are also nutraceuticals that manage it.

The second step is to start drinking two ounces of raw, organic apple cider vinegar every day. You can drink it straight or dilute it in water and sip on it throughout the day. This daily cocktail helps stimulate the production of HCL. The third step to reversing hypochlorhydria is taking a high-quality digestive enzyme supplement after every meal. I use and recommend EnzymixPro (K99) from Apex Energetics. EnzymixPro (K-99) not only helps maintain optimal stomach acid but also supports gallbladder, liver, and pancreatic function.

When your hypochlorhydria is reversed, you can expect your body to run a whole lot more efficiently. After you eat, you should feel nothing other than a sense of fullness. If you're having symptoms after you eat, something in the digestive tract may be malfunctioning. You shouldn't feel sleepy, tired, or sluggish, have gas, belch, or get acid reflux. Those things are common for unhealthy people but not normal. Once digestion is happening properly, our body becomes much more efficient at doing its job and healing itself.

Next comes a cascade effect of improvements in your life. In fact, you may feel so good that you surprise yourself and your loved ones. Once your gut is healed, you are less likely to experience depression, anxiety, excess fatigue, and headaches. Inflammation should go down, chronic pain should go away, and blood sugar should be regulated. Your focus, attention, and concentration should be optimized. You see, living life with these symptoms is like looking through dirty glasses. We get used to it over time, and it's not until you take those glasses off and clean them that you realize how blurry of a view you had. These aren't easy, "take a pill and fix it immediately" solutions. You need the help of a professional functional medicine doctor to guide you through this healing process. Now that we've addressed the elephant in your stomach, let's talk about the next place you can support your gut-brain connection: your microbiome.

CHAPTER TEN

THE MICROBIOME

*Too many of us are not living our dreams
because we are living in our fears.*

—Les Brown

WHAT IS THE HUMAN MICROBIOME?

Discovered in the 1840s but not widely studied or talked about until the 1990s, the microbiome is the most important organ you've probably never heard about. Its role in our bodies is vital and complex. In this chapter, we're going to define the microbiome, understand where it's located and what it does, and talk about ways we can support it and help it flourish.

Our microbiome is made up of trillions of bacteria, viruses, fungi, and other microscopic living things, over a thousand species in total. These little guys are referred to as microorganisms (microbes), hence the name "microbiome." Most of the microbes in your gut live in a pocket of your large intestine called your cecum, and they are collectively called the "gut microbiome." We have ten times the number of microbes in our gut as we have cells in our body. In total, this microbiome weighs between three and five pounds, and it also communicates with our brains via the vagus nerve.

The bacteria in the microbiome help digest our food (especially fiber), regulate our immune system, protect against other bacteria that cause disease, and produce vitamins. One of those is vitamin B12, which is a cofactor in DNA synthesis and aids in amino and fatty acid metabolism. Another is thiamine (vitamin B1) which helps to turn food into energy and keep the nervous system healthy. Then there's riboflavin (vitamin B2), which is important for body growth, helps in red blood cell production, and aids in the release of energy from protein. Finally, there's vitamin K, which is needed for blood coagulation and affects your weight and your brain health.

Without the gut microbiome, it would be impossible to survive. This colonization of microbes starts from the time you're born. Vaginal birth (baby picks up mom's microbes while going through the birth canal) and breastmilk are crucial for establishing a healthy microbiome. As you get older, your microbiome becomes more diversified, and higher microbiome diversity is considered good for your health.

As Healthline.com states, "The microbiome is to our gut health like breathing/oxygen is to our lungs. This is the next generation of health care. We can't live without either one."

When the microbiome is healthy and everything is functioning properly, you easily digest your food without gas, bloating, belching, diarrhea, or constipation. Your digestion is seamless and totally unnoticeable. Your mental health is also in tip-top shape. You may experience less anxiety, depression, or insomnia. You may also notice less joint pain or unexplainable fatigue. Sounds like a wonderful life, right?

We start seeing things go wrong when the microbiome isn't cared for or acknowledged. The three biggest causes of an unhealthy gut microbiome are 1) antibiotic use, 2) the standard American diet and lifestyle, and 3) hypochlorhydria.

The gut microbiome is a balancing act. Fungi, yeast, and bacteria all live together in a cohesive environment, and antibiotics disrupt that ecosystem because they kill the good bugs along with the bad ones. When this happens, fungi like candida (a naturally occurring kind of yeast in the gut) grows out of control and inhibits the large intestine from doing its job. This overgrowth of yeast can grow backward through our digestive system, reaching all the way into our mouths. If you stick out your tongue and it's covered in a thin, white film, that's a sign of candida overgrowth. Often just referred to as "candida," this imbalance damages the gut's ability to digest food properly, which often leads to weight gain, anxiety, depression, and bloating.

I mentioned earlier that the largest concentration of the microbiome lives in the cecum. Next to the cecum is an important sphincter known as the ileocecal valve. This crucial valve is the gateway between the ileum (the last part of the small intestine) and the colon (the first portion of the large intestine), and its job is to allow digested food materials to pass from the small intestine into your large intestine. When this valve malfunctions, things literally "go backward," and bacteria that should be in the colon backs up into the small intestine due to ileocecal valve failure. This condition is known as small intestinal bacterial overgrowth (SIBO). It's a serious problem that can cause major bloating, distension, and discomfort.

The ileocecal valve is supposed to be a one-way valve that only lets food products pass from the small intestine to the large, so what causes it to malfunction? Vagus nerve damage, gluten exposure, inflammation, hypochlorhydria, and gastric surgery can all stress this important sphincter. Yes, the ileocecal valve is controlled by your friend and mine, the vagus nerve.

I've been in practice since 2001, and one of the most commonly overlooked areas with patients suffering from chronic health issues such as brain fog, focus problems, depression, anxiety, insomnia, chronic pain, chronic fatigue, fibromyalgia, headaches, peripheral neuropathy, and small intestinal bacterial overgrowth is the gut-brain/brain-gut axis. If you're dealing with a chronic disease, especially something like anxiety or depression, how many doctors have asked about your gut health? I'm willing to guess the answer is zero.

The gut-brain connection is so incredibly powerful and the health of all three parts—brain, gut, and vagus nerve, affects our entire bodies in ways that most traditional doctors don't acknowledge. I see things differently. Instead of looking at our bodies as many independent organs and systems, I see it as a holistic system. So when I have a patient complaining of joint pain and experiencing depression, I look at the whole human, not just the areas with symptoms. For you to have truly vibrant health, all these systems have to work together seamlessly, and the vagus nerve is the path that connects them all. If one part above fails, it's a domino effect that causes a cascade of dysfunction down through the rest of the system.

MICROBIOME SOLUTIONS

How can we support our microbiome and the trillions of organisms that comprise it? Here are four simple steps you can start taking today for a healthier gut.

1) Limit the use of antibiotics. Overuse of antibiotics is one of the most common destroyers of a healthy gut

microbiome. However, please consult with your doctor before changing your medications.

2) Stop eating a standard American diet and living a standard American lifestyle.

3) Start taking a high-quality probiotic, and add fermented foods like yogurt, kombucha, kimchi, and sauerkraut to your diet. We want to support the microbiome with additional good bacteria, and both of these methods accomplish that goal.

4) Start doing regular vagus nerve exercises (see pages 93–94 in my first book, *License to Heal*).

The most important thing I want you to take away from this chapter is that what you put in your mouth has to be absorbed and assimilated to be beneficial to your brain, body, and gut. If we continually live a lifestyle that damages our gut-brain connection, pretty soon it won't matter what we eat because our bodies won't absorb it anyway. An example of this is the name brand antacid Tums marketing a version of their product with added calcium. Tums make your stomach so basic (aka alkaline) that your body can't absorb the extra calcium anyhow. An acidic stomach is required to break down and absorb vitamins and minerals.

Like the ABCs to Health in Chapter Six, the steps to care for your gut microbiome aren't complicated or fancy, but they do require commitment and consistency. When we get the fundamentals of health right, our gut-brain connection can thrive and our bodies can heal. Can you see a future where your chronic health problems don't hold you back from living the life you desire? I can! In the next chapter, we're going to talk about a plan to accomplish exactly that kind of vision.

CHAPTER ELEVEN

THE STANDARD BARLOW DIET

When you know what you want, and you want it bad enough, you'll find a way to get it.

—Jim Rohn

YOUR PLAN MOVING FORWARD

Now that you understand the gut-brain connection and how it impacts nearly every area of your health, it's time to make a plan of action. You can build the optimal lifestyle and develop habits that will support and promote a healthy gut-brain connection, and these changes can completely change your life. Yes, change is hard. Commitment and discipline are hard. Do you know what else is hard? Waking up in pain every day. Struggling with crippling depression and anxiety. Being overweight. Those things are hard too. It's time to "choose your hard." One path offers hope. What is the other offering you? Declining health? A lackluster future? Choose your hard.

PRINCIPLES OF THE PLAN

1. You don't have to like every change, but you do need to love the results. You may not enjoy every step of this process, but again, what's your alternative? Life at an

8–10 pain level? Is that really the quality of life you're looking for?

2. Define your goal. What is your goal? Be honest with yourself, and take some time to write down where you are now and where you want to go. If this plan could get you as close to a pain level of 1 as possible, would you do it? Would you make those changes to live a vibrant, healthy life again?

3. Embrace this principle: if you create a positive mindset, take positive actions, and maintain positive habits, you will likely reap positive results. If you create a negative mindset, take negative actions and maintain bad habits, you'll likely reap bad results. We live in a sowing and reaping world. What you put into this plan is what you'll get out of it.

Imagine someone who is financially bankrupt comes to you and asks, "What can I do to get my finances back on track?"

Hopefully you'd answer, "Stop spending more than you're earning." Being bankrupt in health is the same way. Stop making the problem worse. Get rid of the bad habits that got you in this predicament and embrace a new way of living.

What is bankrupting your health? After reading this book, you know that the standard American diet and lifestyle are huge contributing factors. You also know that unaddressed past trauma can be contributing factors too, but now you're empowered and educated. You can make these changes! Take what you've learned in this book and start applying that knowledge. Start making deposits in your health bank account.

As my final encouragement to you, if you read this whole book and only make three changes, these are the three I hope you embrace:

1) Stop eating the standard American diet. Kick the high fructose corn syrup, hydrogenated oils, excess sugar, processed carbs, and nutrient-devoid food to the curb, and never let it back in your home. Start eating whole, unprocessed fruits and vegetables. Eat real meats and healthy fats.

2) Stop living the standard American lifestyle by sitting on the couch and numbing your emotions with a screen. Start walking outside, every day if possible. Take time to breathe deeply and fill your lungs with oxygen. Allow your mind ten silent minutes to focus on positive thoughts and wander away from the stressors of day-to-day life.

3) Completely eliminate gluten and casein from your diet. They are detrimental to your long-term health.

I know these changes may seem daunting, but I am doing these things right alongside you. I'm not a rebel without a cause who wants to make your life inconvenient, boring, or difficult. My family and I have personally seen and felt the positive effects of living this way. I'm leading from the front and doing far and above what I'm asking you to do in this book. There's a reason I'm fifty-eight years old, take zero prescription medications, and have a healthy, vibrant life.

As your friend and doctor, I implore you to take responsibility for your life and health and stop taking advice from people who have no idea what they are talking about. Set goals and write out a vision of the life you dream about. Once you have that goal, you can get through the tough moments when you don't want to execute the process. We all have days where we want to sit on the sofa and eat chips, but that's not the recipe for great health and a great life. Your legacy is too important to be wasted on the couch eating chips. You matter more than that, and as long as you're here and breathing, God isn't done with you. You have a purpose and a mission on this earth. If you want to reclaim your life from chronic disease, I'm ready to help. I'm here to help patients who want their life back, and by healing your brain, gut, and vagus nerve, you'll ultimately heal your body and reclaim your life.

PART THREE

MOVING FORWARD TODAY

The following section is an excerpt from Dr. Barlow's first book, *License To Heal: What To Do When Traditional Medicine Has Failed*. Using the 7 Keys To Health, Dr. Barlow walks you through simple and effective changes you can start making today to help you drastically improve the quality of your life. To purchase this best-selling book, please visit www. amazon.com/License-Heal-Traditional-Medicine-Failed.

CHAPTER TWELVE

HOW EXAMS HELP
YOU HEAL

WHAT IS AN EXAM?

In our clinic, every patient's journey begins with a thorough functional neurological exam. This is a head-to-toe neurological evaluation on you. We do this because we treat every single person as a unique, one-of-a-kind case. Think of the way a detective picks up the trail of a murder case that's gone cold. That's how we approach each person's tangled web of dysfunction. The exam is like cracking open that file and looking at every piece of evidence in a new light.

Many times, exams are used more as a "check off" list for doctors. They're such a rich opportunity for the doctor to gather valuable data about their patient, yet they don't bother to ask enough questions or get the right kind of data needed to really solve the patient's problems. Too often, doctors come in with preconceived notions and they don't put their hands on their patients (yes, you actually have to touch your patient to do a neurological exam).

In my experience, performing a thorough neurological exam is both an art and a science. The art aspect focuses on how to perform the exam fluidly and in a systematic way that identifies which systems are not functioning properly and are likely damaged. It's also an art form to identify and then assist the most devastated areas of the patient's brain. The science portion comes from all the neurology in classroom learning at the universities as well as textbooks. Most doctors can do the science part. It's the art part that's rare.

I use the same acronym to guide me through every single patient exam, and it's called POPQRST.

P – Primary complaint. What health issue is having the biggest negative impact on their life? Has anyone else in their family had this issue before?

O – Onset. When did the symptoms start? And is the primary complaint staying the same or getting worse?

P – Pain. What provokes the pain and what makes it better?

Q – Quality of pain. Is there burning, numbness, or tingling?

R – Radiate. Does the pain radiate out or does it stay local?

S – Severity. Rank the pain on a scale of 1–10. How bad is it?

T – Time. What time of day or night is the primary complaint worse?

During this exam, we also test the patient's oxygen levels to determine if they're anemic or not. The body can't heal unless it has the proper supply of oxygen, so this is a crucial first step. We also take their blood pressure (which gives us another hint about their oxygen levels), draw blood and perform intensive blood work, and do glucose testing. All of these tests are getting baseline measurements on the patient's seven keys to health because these keys provide the clues I use to untangle their web of dysfunction and heal their chronic health problems.

During the neurological testing portion of the exam, I use a tuning fork to test the sensitivity of their nervous system. I take the tuning fork, place it on their sternum, and allow them to feel the vibration. That vibration represents a value of 10 and serves as our reference point. Then, I do the same thing but put the tuning fork against their big toe, their thumbs and their shoulders.

Next I do a 2-point discrimination test where I make sure the radial nerve (the nerve which controls sensation in the back of the arm and forearm) is intact and functioning. Then, I test the lower extremities using a two point discrimination test. I check the L-4 saphenous nerve (controls sensation to the inside of the lower leg) and L-5 superficial peroneal nerve (controls the outside of the lower leg). I follow that test with the digit span test where I evaluate the Median nerve which controls the thumb and first and second fingers. I then check Ulnar nerve sensation to part of the ring finger and little finger. Next, I perform the digit span test on the toes via the L-5 superficial peroneal nerve which controls all sensation on the top of the feet as well as all toes (except the small toe which is controlled by the S-1 sural nerve). These tests give me a good indication of how the patient's peripheral nervous system as well as the parietal lobe, located in the back half of the brain, is functioning. Next, I test their reflexes which tells me how well their motor reflexes are responding. Human beings have 10 motor reflexes, and I test all reflexes to see how well their cerebellum, brain and spinal cord are working.

CEREBELLUM TESTS

After that, I ask them to stand up, if they can, and put their feet together and close their eyes. Next, I'll ask the patient to close their eyes and put their right foot in front of the left foot. Then, I have them switch legs. I follow that exercise up by asking them to alternately lift each leg off the ground and hold it at a 90 degree angle. If your cerebellum is functioning optimally you should be able to maintain each balance/ stability test for fifteen seconds. I continue the neurological part of the exam by testing them for smell, fine motor skills, and many more factors that show me the state of their neurological health.

Finger to nose test: I ask the patient to close their eyes and try to place their little finger on the tip of their nose. Fingertip to nose tip. If they miss, they probably have a decreased functioning cerebellum on the side being tested.

It's important to approach an exam with humility and curiosity because I'm working in the field of probabilities, not absolutes. If you're aspiring to be an accountant or an engineer and seeking absolute answers, this probably is not the field for you. Practically nothing in neurology is absolute. Approaching the patient as if they're a completely new, one-of-a-kind case is the most important mental shift I make every time I prepare to do an exam.

THE FUNDAMENTALS OF AN EFFECTIVE EXAM

When a patient comes into the clinic for an exam, they'll have already filled out their paperwork and we have their blood work results on hand. I start the exam by asking them some questions. Then I move into the primary pillars of executing a great exam.

> Pillar One: Where is the problem? Is it neurological, metabolic or both?
>
> Pillar Two: How much can we stimulate the system before it fatigues?
>
> Pillar Three: Do I think I can improve this patient's well being?

Often, the exam reveals new and insightful information that helps us "crack the case." One of my favorite stories is of a young lady who came into the clinic for an exam. She was twenty-one years old and had been a soccer player before her condition forced her to quit sports and drop out of school. She was afflicted with 15–20 seizures per day and had been to all of the major hospitals and experts in the country, yet she was still struggling. Any kind of major stimulation sent her into a seizing fit. If she got out of the car and the sun hit her eyes wrong, she started seizing.

Through neurological testing and the exam, I discovered she had a possible autoimmune disorder, and her oxygen levels were very low. Her feet and hands were also very cold which meant they weren't getting adequate oxygen. It turned out she had developed autoimmunity against her gut.

I prescribed a treatment plan of Vagal nerve stimulation, the 90 day brain and body detox, brain stimulation therapy, and many other home-based modalities. Once we identified the root cause of her problem, which was the autoimmune condition, we began this treatment protocol that targeted the root cause of her dysfunction. Within four months, she no longer had any seizures. Since then, she re-enrolled in school and wants to become a physical therapist. This is the power of doing the right kind of exam. The clues I found in the neurological exam helped me figure out what part of the body was malfunctioning, and when we addressed the root of the problem, she got her life back.

Another favorite story is of a patient who had been told he needed to move to an assisted living facility because of his poor health and lack of coordination. He initially came in for "frozen" shoulders that wouldn't move his arms above 90 degrees. Through a neurological exam, we discovered the part of the brain that was malfunctioning. We used brain stimulation therapy to activate certain muscle groups to reset the neurological receptors in that part of the body which allowed the brain to recognize and execute the full range of motion. Within four minutes of his first treatment, he went from being able to lift his arms from 90 degrees to lifting them above his head to 180 degrees. From that point, we worked together to heal a whole cascade of chronic health problems that were holding him back and limiting his quality of life. Within nine months of receiving treatment at our clinic, he and his family were back to adventuring. They've since traveled to Yellowstone National Park, Israel, and taken many other big trips.

This is why I treat every single person as a unique, one-of-a-kind case. Every person's tangled web of dysfunction is different and caused by a different combination of dysfunctional processes. The exam is how we open that cold-case file and start to uncover what's going on beneath the surface.

CHAPTER THIRTEEN

OUR PROGRAM

THE PHASES OF DECLINE

The "phases of decline" refer to the stages someone struggling with chronic health problems will experience as their dysfunctional process advances. While this book is ultimately about hope and the encouragement that it is often possible to stop and reverse physical damage and disorders, you also need to take these phases of decline seriously because there is a point of no return. At this point, the body becomes so damaged that it's not possible to regenerate your health to a normal state. Let's take a look at the phases of decline for the three most common maladies I see in my clinic—brain disorders, knee pain, and neuropathy.

PHASES OF DECLINE FOR BRAIN DISORDERS

Phase One: Full Health

No symptoms expressed at all.

Phase Two: Easily Dismissable Symptoms

These are things like brain fog that just won't go away, difficulty focusing and concentrating for long periods of time, and a loss of attention to the things you normally enjoy and love. At this point, your brain cells are actually dying, yet most people won't take action, instead choosing to casually dismiss the changes. The patient usually doesn't take responsibility or action, at least not yet.

Phase Three/Four: Recognizable Symptoms

At this stage, things are beginning to progress. You may walk into a room and forget why you walked in there in the first place. Or you may call someone on the phone and forget why you called them. This is an advanced stage of brain degeneration. This is the point where the adult kids may tease their parents about having "old timers" syndrome or say things like "Mom is just losing it." At this stage, it's very important to filter who you listen to. Your healthcare provider, your kids, your friends, or your spouse may laugh it off, but it's nothing to joke about. At this phase, you must stand up and take responsibility for your health. If you know something isn't right, keep pursuing a solution until you get answers.

Phase Five: The Limitation of Matter

At this stage, the brain is degenerated to the point where the person is no longer motivated and simply doesn't have the brain ability to solve their own problems. They no longer see themselves as the problem; instead, everyone else has a problem. When someone reaches this stage, it is very hard and nearly impossible to bring them back. It's a very serious case when someone gets to this stage. It's called "limitation of matter" because at this point, the brain has degenerated so far that it's unable to regenerate and repair to its former state. I don't accept patients for care who are at this stage of degeneration.

Common Treatments For Brain Disorders

These are the common in-clinic treatments that I do for brain-based disorders.

- Clear Mind neurofeedback program – this tool instantly and non-invasively identifies brain dysfunction. I use these results to know which areas of the brain to stimulate to help it begin functioning optimally again.
- Exercise with oxygen therapy – This is simply putting an oxygen mask on the patient and having them ride a stationary bike for twenty minutes while breathing in pure oxygen.
- Hako-Med – This powerful machine helps stimulate proper nerve function.
- Pulse Electro-Magnetic Field (PEMF) machine – This machine is like a battery re-charger for your body. It helps to recharge the cells of the body to the perfect charge to maintain optimal cellular function.
- At-Home Exercises – Vagal stimulation exercises, 90 day brain and body detox, and proper nutritional supplementation.

PHASES OF DECLINE FOR KNEE PAIN

I classify chronic knee pain as anything that has existed for three months or longer. Most of the people who come see me for knee pain have had it for years, if not decades, and can barely walk or get out of a chair. They often have difficulty getting out of bed or off the couch, and their life is severely impacted by their pain. One of the first things I do with every knee pain patient is take a radiograph (x-rays) of the knee. We can use regenerative medicine at the clinic, but in order for that treatment to be effective, there has to be a space between the knee joint as seen on the radiograph. The space is important because it means there is still tissue present that can be rehabilitated. If there's no space, they've reached the limitation of matter and have to be referred out for a knee replacement. I don't accept everyone that comes into the office as a patient. If I do the exam and based on their results I don't think I can help them, I refer the patient to a health professional who I think can help.

However, if the radiograph shows enough spacing in the joint, I may start with a regenerative medicine treatment plan to help them eliminate their chronic pain and regain mobility. Here are some of the solutions that have worked exceptionally well for our knee pain patients.

Common Treatments For Knee Pain

- The Ergo-Flex Knee-On-Track – This is a machine that decompresses the knee and opens up the joint space, promoting healing and pain relief.
- Oxygen therapy with exercise – I talked about this treatment earlier in the book, but this is simply putting

an oxygen mask on the patient and having them ride a stationary bike for twenty minutes while breathing in oxygen.

- Hako-Med – This powerful machine helps stimulate proper nerve function.
- Laser therapy – This treatment decreases inflammation and pain by dilating the capillaries to promote blood flow and encourage the healing properties to access the joint.
- Pulse Electro-Magnetic Field (PEMF) machine – This machine is like a battery re-charger for your body. It helps to recharge the cells of the body to the perfect charge to maintain optimal cellular function.
- Trigenics – This modality activates the two main receptors of the brain so that they fire into the cerebellum, spinal cord and brain to decrease pain and increase mobility.

PHASES OF DECLINE FOR NEUROPATHY

Neuropathy patients are usually the most complicated cases because neuropathy can be caused by so many different dysfunctions. These patients often have oxygen problems, glucose problems, and their brain has deteriorated because of a lack of stimulation from their feet. Many people with neuropathy also have erectile or sexual dysfunction.

Phase One: The feet begin tingling or experiencing a pins and needles sensation.

Phase Two: Coldness and color changes in the toes and feet.

Phase Three: The tingling becomes a burning pain.

Phase Four: Loss of sensation in the legs, feet, toes.

Common Treatments For Neuropathy

- Blood sugar regulation – I work with the patient to help them balance their blood sugar so their neurological system can stabilize and begin the work of healing.

- Spinal decompression – Many patients with neuropathy have L5 damage so I use decompression therapy to relieve the pressure on that area of the spine.

- Oxygen therapy with exercise – I talked about this treatment earlier in the book, but this is simply putting an oxygen mask on the patient and having them ride a stationary bike for twenty minutes while breathing in oxygen.

- Hako-Med on their feet – This powerful machine helps stimulate proper nerve function.

- Laser therapy – This treatment decreases inflammation and pain by dilating the capillaries to promote blood flow and encourage the healing properties to access the joint.

- Pulse Electro-Magnetic Field (PEMF) machine – This machine is like a battery re-charger for your body. It helps to recharge the cells of the body to the perfect charge to maintain optimal cellular function.

- Trigenics – This modality activates the two main receptors of the brain so that they fire into the cerebellum, spinal cord and brain to decrease pain and increase mobility.

- Clear Mind neurofeedback program – this tool instantly and non-invasively identifies brain dysfunction. I use these results to know which areas of the brain to stimulate to help it start functioning optimally again.

- At-Home Exercises – Brain-Body-Gut 90 day detox and proper nutritional supplementation.

CUSTOM MADE

A truly custom, one-of-a-kind healthcare program will impact your health in a way you've never experienced before because it is created uniquely for you. I don't accept everyone for care. If someone isn't fully committed, they're too neurologically damaged, or they're too far degenerated, I'm not going to take them for care and waste their time or money. When I accept someone for care, I make them a promise that I'm on this journey with them, and we're in it to win it. I will exhaust every option I know in order to optimize their recovery. However, we both need to have realistic expectations. If their expectations are beyond what I can give them, we need to realign. I'm always going to under promise and over deliver, and sometimes tough love requires telling people the truth that they don't want to hear.

A custom healthcare program to heal your chronic disease always comes as a result of a thorough and effective neurological examination process, and it always addresses all aspects of your metabolic and neurological health. However, the truth is that if they don't follow the program I prescribe them, they're probably not going to get the results they want. No one is going to care more about your health than you. If you don't want to be well, live vibrantly, and leave a legacy, no one is going to do it for you. I'm totally committed to the patient, but they need to be "all in" too.

CHAPTER FOURTEEN

OUR PARTNERSHIP

THE ULTIMATE PARTNERSHIP

A successful relationship between a doctor and a patient is founded in truth, commitment, and trust. When both doctor and patient are totally committed to the healing process, there's no limit to the chronic problems that can be solved.

When I see patients who are totally committed to healing, the one thing they all have in common is a belief that they are valuable. They see themselves as created in the image of God and believe that they're worth putting in the work, making the changes, and spending the time and money to find true healing. Do you see yourself as a valuable person? Are you willing to take responsibility for your life? Are you willing to do what it takes outside of the office to optimize your recovery? If you answered yes to all of these questions, then you may be a fit for care at my clinic.

There's no way that someone can read this book and think I'm lukewarm about the commitment it takes to change your life. Why would I have gone through everything I've overcome to "kind of" do this half way? I had to spend years of my life and tens of thousands of dollars to reach this point in my career where I could help the toughest of the tough cases. Why would I dabble or give this a half-hearted effort? No way! I won't do it. I'm asking you to step up and do for yourself what I've done for myself. Look at your life and where you want to go, then make a plan and get after it.

A successful doctor and patient relationship has to be built on truth. I see a lot of people who want their doctor to be fully committed but they don't want to be all in. Everyone says they're committed until they realize they have to take responsibility. I can only be responsible for me and my actions. The patient has to believe, "I am worth this. I am worth the time, effort, and money it takes to return me to my full potential because I have something valuable to give this world." Some people die twenty years before they're put in the ground, but I believe it's possible to age and never act "old." Getting older is inevitable, but being old is optional.

I want to have such a great doctor and patient relationship that when the treatment plan comes to fruition and you get the results you wanted, you are so excited that you want to give a testimonial or refer a friend to the clinic. If that happens, I know my team and I are doing a good job. In order for that to happen, both parties have to be on the same page, with common timelines and expectations.

I don't accept everyone for care at this clinic. If you come in, do an exam, and I accept you for care, there is hope. Even if you've heard "no" from other doctors, or been told that "you're just going to have to learn to live with it," there still may be hope. How many doctors have talked to you about anemia? About your blood sugar levels? About autoimmune conditions or gut health? So many medical doctors keep trying to put the proverbial duct tape over the check engine light, but it simply doesn't work. You can't keep covering up what the body is trying to tell you.

There is hope and life change is possible. It is possible to be healed from chronic issues, if they are caught early enough. It is possible to untangle your web of dysfunction, but I can't do it by myself. I can't help you unless you're also willing to help yourself. If you're willing to put in the work, I'm not going to stop until I get you results.

Want more from *License To Heal*? Order today at www. amazon.com/License-Heal-Traditional-Medicine-Failed.

Are you living each day with chronic pain? Have you been told that there's no hope for a solution and you're "just going to have to learn to live with it?" Most people (and their doctors) don't understand the root of chronic health problems, but Dr. Andy Barlow is here to help unravel the often mysterious causes of chronic pain. A chronic symptom is like the check engine light flashing in your car. It alerts you to the problem but doesn't tell you where it's coming from. The good news is that it's possible to untangle your web of dysfunction and find the root cause of your chronic pain. Using his 7 Keys to Health, Dr. Barlow walks you through simple and effective changes that you can start making today that will help you drastically improve the quality of your life. Dr. Barlow is a chiropractor, functional medicine doctor, and neurological specialist who earned his diplomate and completed a fellowship through the elite Carrick Institute and has since taught hundreds of doctors from around the world this life-changing material. At his clinic in Tupelo, Mississippi, he specializes in helping people that traditional medicine has failed. If you are ready to heal, take this life-changing journey with Dr. Barlow. With his characteristic wit and emphasis on taking personal responsibility for your health, he teaches you his 7 Keys to Health and helps you untangle your unique web of chronic dysfunction.

ABOUT THE AUTHOR

Dr. Barlow has been in private practice in Tupelo, MS since June 2001. He is a national and international lecturer and educator in the area of Functional Neurology. Dr. Barlow is the lead U.S. instructor for the Trigenics Institute as well as the American Functional Neurology Institute. Dr. Barlow is a Board-Certified Chiropractic Neurologist and a Fellow of the American College of Functional Neurology. Dr. Andy Barlow is a graduate of Pontotoc High School, Itawamba Community College, and received his doctorate in chiropractic at Life University in Marietta, GA. He served four years in the U.S. Navy, stationed in Great Lakes, IL, Yokosuka, Japan on board the aircraft carrier USS Midway CV-41 as well as aircraft carrier in Coronado, CA on board the USS Constellation CV-64.

Dr. Barlow received his honorable discharge from the U.S. Navy June 1986. To contact Dr. Barlow, please call him and his team at the Chiropractic Neurology Center of Tupelo at 662.844.1414 or email Dr. Barlow at askdrbarlow_afni@ yahoo.com.

MORE TESTIMONIALS
OF HEALING

"When I first came to Dr. Barlow's clinic in May 2021, I was using a walker to get around and in extreme pain in the lower back, right hip, and right leg. I had been to several neurologists, had shots in the back, and a nerve block. None of it helped the problem, so they sent me to pain management. They just wanted to give me more prescriptions, but I didn't want any more drugs. I had heard other people talk about Dr. Barlow's clinic, so I decided to give him a try. Within one month of coming to Dr. Barlow's clinic, I had no pain in my hip or leg and started walking with a cane instead of a walker. I still have some lower back pain, but that has improved a lot. He did bloodwork and tests that no other doctor had ever thought of doing. I did their detox program and supplements. Dr. Barlow has helped tremendously. I am now walking without a cane, am standing up straighter, and have more energy. I want to thank Dr. Barlow and all the staff for helping me. I would highly recommend Dr. Barlow to anyone that traditional medicine has failed."

—Jim Miller

"I saw an ad on the television where a lady with digestive issues said that Dr. Barlow did extensive blood work on her. I made an appointment, got the lab work done, and got an x-ray on my shoulder that I had strained two years prior. While we waited for the lab results to come back, Dr. Barlow started to do therapies on my shoulder. Within minutes of this treatment, my arm felt better, and I had a wider range of motion.

After listening to me describe my major reason for the office visit, he suspected that I had a leaky gut. He recommended that I get off gluten, eggs, and dairy. He put me on a detox program to help heal my leaky gut. It was amazing! Within two days, my complexion began to clear, and my liver stopped aching. Yes, the liver does ache even though a specialist told me that it does not.

When the lab results came back, I learned I have a plethora of issues that stem from the leaky gut. Instead of being shocked and dismayed, I felt enlightened. Now we knew what the problem was, and I could start the healing process. In essence, it was like the first day of the rest of my life.

I thank God for Dr. Barlow. He is a caring and highly intelligent person who wants to get to the root of the problem instead of writing a prescription and putting a bandage on it. Needless to say, I highly recommend Dr. Barlow, especially if you are having any type of bodily issues that haven't been addressed to your satisfaction. He and his staff are result oriented, and they work diligently to meet your health needs."

—M.W. patient

"My husband and I both have been patients of Dr. Barlow since August 2021. We were dealing with issues that had either been misdiagnosed or not addressed in depth. Since being introduced to methods that bring healing, we have both begun to recover from neuropathy, back pain, and gut issues. The therapy injections, supplements, and overall healthy eating habits have brought us back not only to having more energy but also have improved our brain function and stomach digestion. Being educated on how to transform our lives has led us to true healing."

—Cliff & Lisa Tubb

"I just completed *License to Heal* and feel like this book was written about me. I'm anxious to get started on the "First Steps" listed on page 91."

—Carrie Hanscom

"I had several friends coming in to see Dr. Barlow. They were getting such good results that I decided to see if he could help me, too. I started coming into Dr. Barlow's clinic in March of 2021. I have had two back surgeries and two knee surgeries in the past. I came in to see Dr. Barlow for lower back pain, leg pain, and pain in my feet. He did blood work and put me on a detox program. I felt so much better after doing the detox, plus I lost weight. Overall, I am doing great! I would recommend anyone go see Dr. Barlow. He cares about your well being, is a great doctor, and he has an amazing staff. I am well pleased with my progress."

—Eddie Key

"I first saw Dr. Barlow on TV and there was just something genuine about him. I didn't think much about it until one day the bulging disc in my neck that I had been previously diagnosed with was bothering me to a point I could no longer stand. When I finally decided after a year or two of physical therapy that I wasn't getting any better, I thought about Dr. Barlow. I guess it was the Lord that led me to go to him. The first day, he did an exam and X-rays and told me he could help me. I wasn't expecting him to start on me right away, but he did. After one treatment of therapy and something else he did by treating my neck, I honestly already felt better and I knew I was in the right place. I did a detox and extensive blood work. A few therapy sessions later, I was a new man! It's been three or four years now and I haven't looked back. Since then, I've had problems in other areas, so I knew what to do and where to go. I recommended him to my wife, now she's going and doing better as well. Dr. Barlow is the real deal and I highly recommend him!"

—John Hogan

"When I first came to Dr. Barlow, I was having a lot of trouble with my chronic back and neck pain from a previous wreck I had been in that had caused a lot of damage. I did a ten-week detox and Dr. Barlow ran an extensive array of bloodwork. After about three weeks into Dr. Barlow's program, I noticed improvement. From then on, I continued to gradually get better. The staff is wonderful. I would recommend anyone and everyone to Dr. Barlow. He truly cares about his patients and their health."

—Marty Wade

DR. BARLOW'S
RECOMMENDED RESOURCES

- **Dr. Barlow's American Functional Neurology Institute – website:** AFNIseminars.com
- **Ergo-Flex:** Back on Track, Knee on Track, Brain & Body O2 – Linda Anderson 936-201-6923
- **Clearmind:** Denise 714-609-7140
- **Shockwave:** Chuck 561-707-0530
- **HakoMed:** Marshall 828-231-7406
- **Trigenics Institute:** 416-481-1936
- Carrickinstitute.com
- courses.functionalneurologyseminars.com – **Instructors:** Dr. Datis Kharrazian & Dr. Brandon Brock

- **Microlight, Inc.:** Mike Barbour 281-433-4648
- **TruDOSE Regenerative Technology:** Connie Esch 508-450-2160, ConnieE@bbiosciences.com

REFERENCES

Suganya, K., & Koo, B.-S. Gut-Brain Axis: Role of Gut Microbiota on Neurological Disorders and How Probiotics/Prebiotics Beneficially Modulate Microbial and Immune Pathways to Improve Brain Functions. *International Journal of Molecular Sciences.* http://www.ncbi.nlm.nih.gov/pmc/articles/PMC7589356/.

Breakthrough study: Gastroenterology 2009

This study identifies an increase in gluten sensitivity in the US. Blood samples were collected from 1948–1954 of 9,000 healthy young adults. The researchers found the prevalence of celiac disease in increased dramatically during the past fifty years, from 1:700 to 1:100.

Kharrazian, Datis. *Why Isn't My Brain Working?: A Revolutionary Understanding of Brain Decline and Effective Strategies to Recover Your Brain's Health.* Carlsbad, CA: Elephant Press, 2013.

Kharrazian, Datis. *Why Do I Still Have Thyroid Symptoms?: When My Lab Tests Are Normal: A Revolutionary Breakthrough in Understanding Hashimoto's Disease and Hypothyroidism.* Carlsbad (CA): Elephant Press, 2010.

~ IN MEMORY OF ~

Dr. David Shreve, DC
Dr. David Chalfant, DC

Made in United States
Orlando, FL
20 January 2024

42729966R10096